Basic Surgical Skills and Techniques

Basic Surgical Skills and Techniques

Second Edition

Editors

Sudhir Kumar Jain
MS FRCS (Edinburgh) FACS FICS
Professor
Department of Surgery
Maulana Azad Medical College
New Delhi, India

David L Stoker
MD FRCS (Edinburgh)
Consultant Surgeon
University College of London Hospitals and
North Middlesex University Hospital
London, UK

Raman Tanwar MS
Consultant Surgeon
Jyoti Hospital
Gurgaon, Haryana, India

JAYPEE BROTHERS MEDICAL PUBLISHERS (P) LTD

New Delhi • London • Philadelphia • Panama

Jaypee Brothers Medical Publishers (P) Ltd

Headquarters

Jaypee Brothers Medical Publishers (P) Ltd
4838/24, Ansari Road, Daryaganj
New Delhi 110 002, India
Phone: +91-11-43574357
Fax: +91-11-43574314
Email: jaypee@jaypeebrothers.com

Overseas Offices

J.P. Medical Ltd
83, Victoria Street, London
SW1H 0HW (UK)
Phone: +44-2031708910
Fax: +02-03-0086180
Email: info@jpmedpub.com

Jaypee Brothers Medical Publishers Ltd
The Bourse
111 South Independence Mall East
Suite 835, Philadelphia, PA 19106, USA
Phone: + 267-519-9789
Email: joe.rusko@jaypeebrothers.com

Jaypee Brothers Medical Publishers (P) Ltd
Shorakhute, Kathmandu, Nepal
Phone: +00977-9841528578
Email: jaypee.nepal@gmail.com

Jaypee-Highlights Medical Publishers Inc.
City of Knowledge, Bld. 237, Clayton
Panama City, Panama
Phone: +507-301-0496
Fax: +507-301-0499
Email: cservice@jphmedical.com

Jaypee Brothers Medical Publishers (P) Ltd
17/1-B Babar Road, Block-B, Shaymali
Mohammadpur, Dhaka-1207
Bangladesh
Mobile: +08801912003485
Email: jaypeedhaka@gmail.com

Website: www.jaypeebrothers.com
Website: www.jaypeedigital.com

Inquiries for bulk sales may be solicited at: jaypee@jaypeebrothers.com

Basic Surgical Skills and Techniques

First Edition: 2008
Second Edition: **2013**

ISBN: 978-93-5090-375-9

Printed at: Ajanta Offset & Packagings Ltd., New Delhi

Dedicated to

Our families,
for their support in spite of their neglection
by us during the process of this work
Our parents, for their blessings
Our teachers, for their wisdom
Our students, who inspire us daily
and
Our patients,
from whom we continue to learn daily

Contributors

Beryl Antoinette De Souza MD
Specialist Plastic Surgeon
Chelsea and Westminister Hospital
London, UK

David L Stoker MD FRCS (Edinburgh)
Consultant Surgeon
University College of London Hospitals and
North Middlesex University Hospital
London, UK

Gemma Conn MD
Specialist Registrar
Department of General Surgery
Colchester General Hospital
London, UK

Raman Tanwar MS
Consultant Surgeon
Jyoti Hospital
Gurgaon, Haryana, India

Sudhir Kumar Jain MS FRCS (Edinburgh) FACS FICS
Professor
Department of Surgery
Maulana Azad Medical College
New Delhi, India

Preface to the Second Edition

The field of surgery is facing an era of rapid modernisation and technical advancements. In this state, it is a challenging task to agglomerate every change that the modern-day surgeon is incorporating into his surgical technique. Thankfully, these new changes have their roots tracing back to the older and established concepts in surgery, which have stood the test of time. Keeping this situation in mind, we have made a humble attempt at incorporating the new advances and keeping this book updated. Apart from thoroughly revising the contents and reflowing the text to enhance readability, and understanding of surgical concepts, four new chapters have been added to cover important topics such as Lasers, Instruments, Basic Surgical Procedures and Newer Devices that we commonly encounter in the operating rooms as surgeons of the modern era. The readers will also notice that the diagrams are now more vivid, accurate and descriptive. We are extremely thankful to readers from all around the globe who have helped us cover what is actually needed by sending us their valuable suggestions. We hope that our readers will find the book valuable and that we will continue to get their constant support and valuable suggestions as before.

Sudhir Kumar Jain
David L Stoker
Raman Tanwar

Preface to the First Edition

Apprentices in surgery need a basic set of practical skills in order to care for their patients well. Although many of these skills are same as those used by their 20th century predecessors, today's trainees need to keep abreast of rapidly changing and advancing technologies that were not available even ten years ago.

At the same time, basic surgical training for medical students and for junior doctors is being compressed into a shorter time frame, as other medical specialities evolve and need to be taught in growing curricula. There is increasing emphasis on communication skills, and self-directed learning in many undergraduate programmes, and the student of surgery today has, therefore, to learn more in less available time. He/she will have less "hands on" experience in theatre, ward or clinic and inevitably the practical aspects of surgery tend to suffer.

This small book aims to facilitate the more rapid learning required in a modern surgical programme, with concise chapters on the main techniques that need to be mastered in the early years of training. It is intended to be read mainly by senior medical students, and housemen or interns, but may also be a useful revision for those about to take their first surgical postgraduate examinations. It is the book written by working general surgeons to enhance the practical training of their own teams. It is also an international collaboration between London and New Delhi, and will be of use to students studying the art and science of surgery everywhere. It is not an exhaustive reference book, but more of a brief guide, to be used as a learning tool mainly in operating theatres and emergency rooms.

It contains simple lists and diagrams with no superfluous text. There are clear explanations which should aid the student from scrubbing up to suturing up. This book is designed to enhance practical training, and the student is encouraged to spend as much time as possible putting the basic skills described to good use in a clinical environment. Surgery remains largely an apprenticeship speciality, where only lots of practice will make perfect.

Sudhir Kumar Jain
David L Stoker

Acknowledgements

Our sincere thanks to Shri Jitendar P Vij (Group Chairman) and Mr Ankit Vij (Managing Director) of M/s Jaypee Brothers Medical Publishers (P) Ltd, New Delhi, India, for the encouragement, support and inspiration. We are grateful to Mr Tarun Duneja (Director-Publishing) for helping us by valuable suggestions during the process of this work. We express our special thanks to the whole production team of Jaypee Brothers Medical Publishers (P) Ltd, especially Mr KK Raman (Production Manager), Mr Subrata Adhikary, Mr Rajesh Sharma, Mr Laxmidhar Padhiary, Mrs Uma Adhikari and Mr Satendra Chand, for their hard work, professionalism and help throughout the process of this publication.

Contents

Scrubbing, Gowning and Gloving Techniques

1

Sudhir Kumar Jain, David L Stoker

SURGICAL HAND SCRUB

A surgical hand scrub is performed prior to donning sterile gown and gloves. Hand scrub does not render the skin sterile, but makes it surgically clean, by reducing the number of organisms, hence reducing the risk to the patient in case a glove is perforated during surgery. Purpose of surgical hand scrub are three fold:

1. To remove transient microorganisms, debris from the skin of hands, forearm and nails.
2. To inhibit the re-growth of microorganisms in between the two procedures.
3. To reduce the resident microorganism counts to the lowest possible level.

Surgical scrub can be defined as systematic washing and scrubbing of the hands and forearms with an effective antibacterial cleaning solution to render the skin free from bacteria as far as possible.

The following two types of bacterial population are normally present on the skin.

Transient Organisms

These organisms are introduced on to the skin surface by soil, dust and by various other substances that come in contact with the skin. Surgical scrub will remove most of these organisms.

Resident Organisms

They are mainly gram-negative and gram-positive bacteria with a natural habitat under the finger nails and in the deeper layers of skin, e.g. in hair follicles, sweat glands and in sebaceous glands. Scrubbing removes bacteria from the skin surface and from just beneath the surface. After gloving, resident bacteria from the deeper layers are brought to the skin surface by perspiration and oily secretions, and the bacterial count on the skin again increases. Hand scrub therefore needs to be repeated between procedures.

Preparation Before Scrubbing

Personal cleanliness is of paramount importance for members of the surgical team. This includes daily showers, frequent shampoos and attention to hands and finger nails. Staff with rashes, infective lesions or open wounds of the skin on hands, nails or arms should not scrub for a procedure. Staff with common cold, sore throats or systemic infections should also not scrub.

Scrubbed personnel should have short nails, such that they are not visible over the tips of the fingers. Short nails are easy to clean and if kept smooth will not puncture the gloves. Finger nails should be free from nail varnish, as chipped fingernail polish can harbor greater numbers of bacteria. Artificial nails should never be worn as fungal growth can occur when moisture becomes trapped between the artificial nail and the natural nail. Skin of the scrubbed personnel should be free from cuts or boils.

Watches, bracelets and rings should be removed and kept in a safe place. Bacteria and dead skin cells accumulate beneath jewellery. Every surgical team member should wear a clean, short sleeved cotton scrub suit before entering the semi-restricted/restricted areas of the surgical suite. Sleeves of the scrub shirt should be four inches above the elbow.

Street clothes or hospital uniforms are not allowed in restricted areas. A scrub shirt should be tucked in to the trousers to avoid contamination by the shirt tail flapping into the sterile field. Trouser legs should not touch the floor as this may transport bacteria from one place to another. Personnel should wear shoes especially assigned for the surgical suite. Shoes should cover the toes completely. This is to prevent injury from sharp or heavy instruments falling from the operating table, and to prevent soiling of toes by the patient's blood or body fluids. Shoes should be cleaned at the end of the day. Street shoes are not allowed in restricted areas unless covered by sterile shoe covers. Shoe covers should be used on a single use basis and must be discarded on leaving the restricted area.

Personnel should wear a disposable surgical cap in such a manner so that hair is covered completely to avoid contamination of the sterile field by falling hair or dandruff (Fig. 1.1).

A surgical mask should be worn by the surgeon, and assistant to cover the nose and mouth completely. This protects the patient from oropharyngeal bacteria exhaled by surgical team members (Fig. 1.1). It may not be necessary to wear a mask for all laparoscopic or endoscopic surgical procedures.

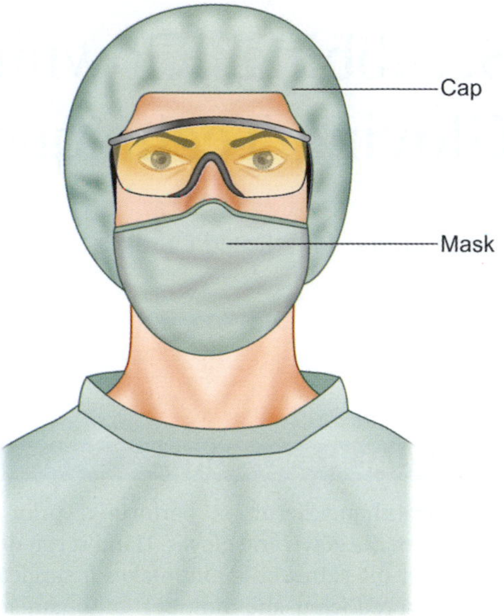

Figure 1.1: Proper method of wearing cap and mask

Environment and Equipment in Scrub Area

The scrub area should be large enough to allow the scrub personnel to gown and glove safely without hindrance. A wall clock should be strategically placed to time the scrub, and there should be provision to control water temperature. Sink height should be sufficient to minimize splashing, and taps should be elbow or knee operated.

Solutions Used

Hibiscrub—(Cholorhexidine 4%)

Betadine scrub—(Povidone iodine 7.5%)

Soap

These solutions are available in a liquid form. The first two are preferred because:

1. They are nonirritating to most people.
2. They leave a minimum number of micro-organisms on the skin.
3. They have a prolonged antibacterial effect on the skin when used regularly. They leave a film on the skin which keeps the resident bacteria to a minimum and do not interfere with the skin's natural resistance to transient bacteria.
4. They lather easily in hot, cold or hard water.
5. The amount of detergent needed is small.

Scrubbing Method

Scrub should be performed before the first case in the morning and then in between cases. Two methods of scrub technique are used, the time method and the brush stroke method. Rinsing time is not included in the total scrub time if the time method is used. In the brush-stroke method, a prescribed number of brush strokes are applied lengthwise to each surface of fingers, hands and arms.

Unsterile objects should not be touched once the scrub process has begun. If this happens accidentally, the entire scrub process should be repeated.

Scrub Up Technique

Scrubbing procedure must take a minimum of two minutes if scrub solutions are used and five minutes if soap is used. Water temperature should be set at a comfortable level. Wet hands and forearms at the start of scrub up (Figs 1.2A and B). Dispense around 5 ml of antibacterial soap solution in to the palm. A nail brush should be used only on nails or in web spaces but not on rest of the skin (Fig. 1.3). Scrubbing should start from fingers to one inch below the elbow, not from the elbow to the fingers (Fig. 1.4). Hands should be held higher than the elbow, so that water flows downwards draining off the elbows (Fig. 1.5). Water splashing on theater clothes should be avoided as wet clothes may cause contamination of the sterile gown. Hands and forearms should be washed and rinsed at least twice after scrubbing (Figs 1.6A and B). Following the final rinse, the hands and forearms should be elevated away from the body allowing water to drop from the elbows. Hands and forearms should be dried using a folded disposable hand towel separately for each side. Drying should start from the fingers going towards the elbows. The towels should be discarded immediately after drying the hands and forearms. Towel should remain folded to double thickness while drying (Figs 1.7 to 1.10).

SURGICAL GOWN TECHNIQUE

Gowns should be properly fitting, permitting adequate freedom of movement. Each sleeve should be provided with a tight fitting cuff. Gowns should ideally be water repellent.

When donning a gown one should touch only the back surface. If the outside of the gown is touched, it is deemed contaminated and should be discarded. Gowns are folded with the back facing the scrubbed person to facilitate sterile gowning.

Scrubbed personnel should keep their hands and arms above their waist and away from the body at an angle of 20 to 30° above the elbows. If scrubbed hands and arms fall below waist level they are considered contaminated.

After donning, the parts which are considered sterile are sleeves (except the axillary area) and the front from waist level to a few inches below the neck opening. Gowns must be made of material that minimises the passage of microorganisms and body fluids, and should also be tear and puncture resistant. They should be lint free to reduce particle dissemination into the wound or the environment.

Procedure for Gowning

Lift the inner or back side of the neck of the gown upwards and away from the table (Fig. 1.11). While holding at the neckline, the gown is allowed to unfold completely with inner side facing the wearer (Fig. 1.12).

Slip both hands into the open armholes keeping the hands at shoulder level and away from the body. Push both hands and forearm into the sleeves of the gown but advance hands up to the proximal edge of the cuff. Do not allow hands to come out of the cuff (Figs 1.13 and 1.14). An ungloved hand should not touch the front of

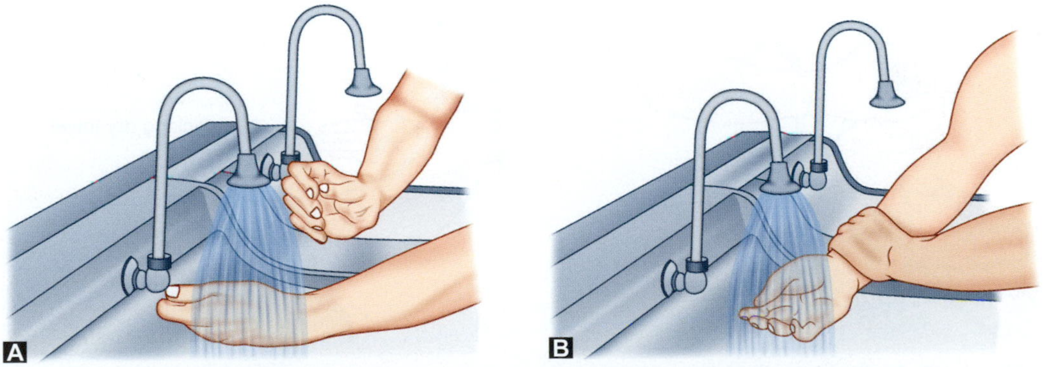

Figures 1.2A and B: Wet hands and forearms before starting scrub up

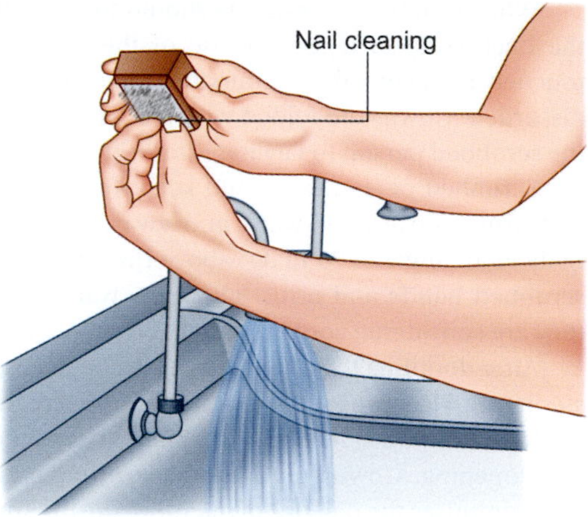

Figure 1.3: Scrub fingernails with nail brush

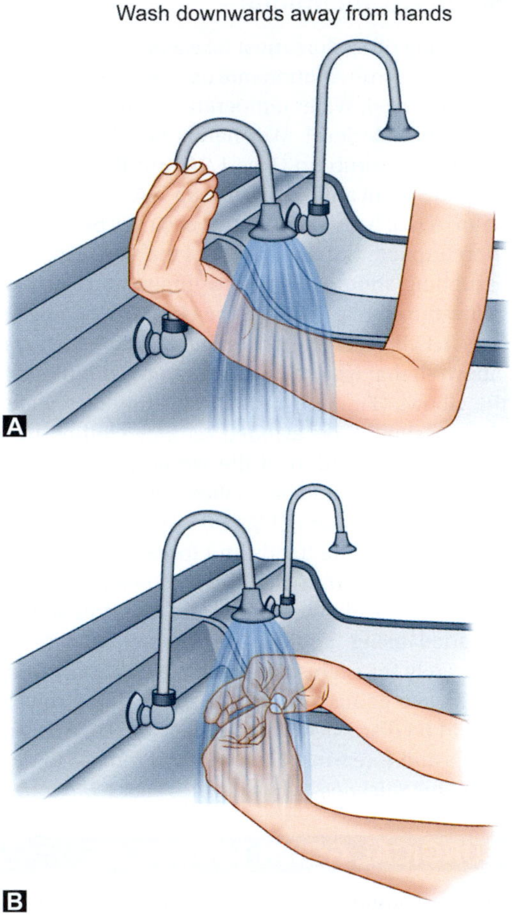

Figures 1.6A and B: Rinsing forearms and hands

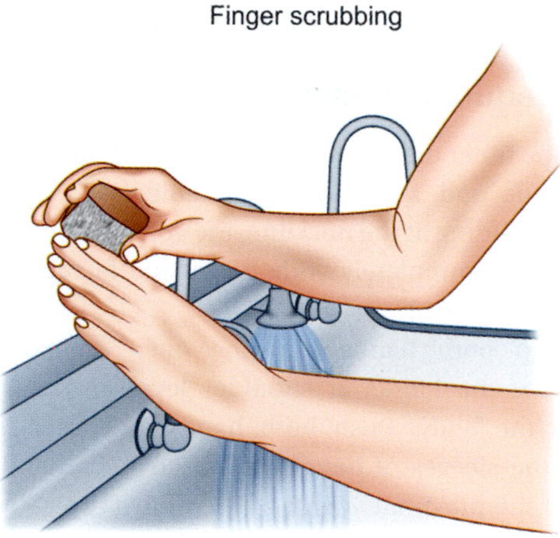

Figure 1.4: Scrub all sides of fingers

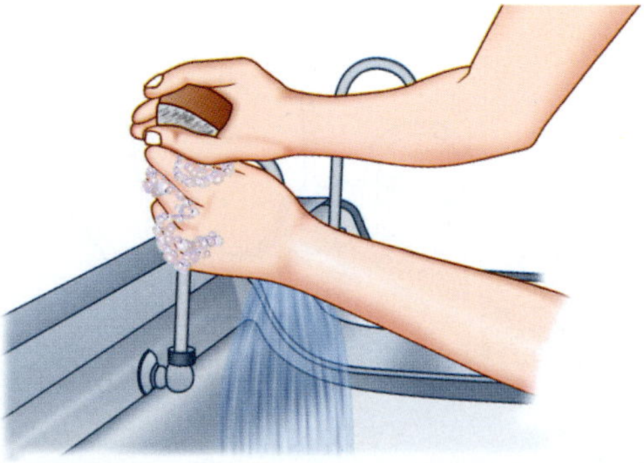

Figure 1.5: Continuing scrub process on hands

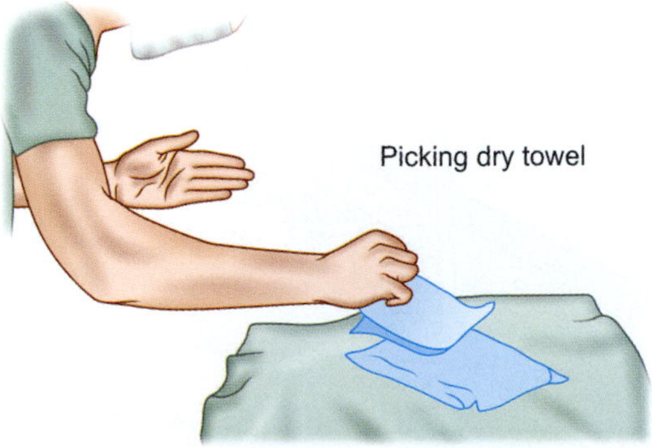

Figure 1.7: Picking up folded hand towel

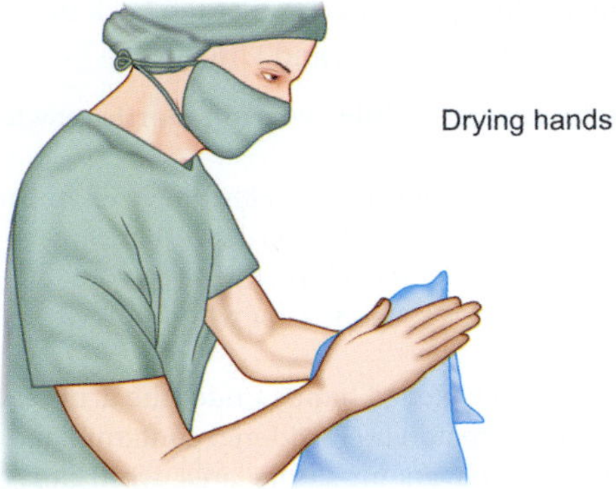

Figure 1.8: Drying the elbows

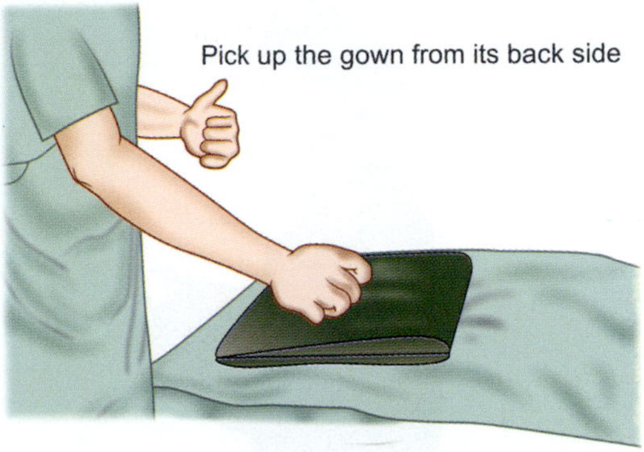

Pick up the gown from its back side

Figure 1.11: Pick up the gown from its inner side near the neck

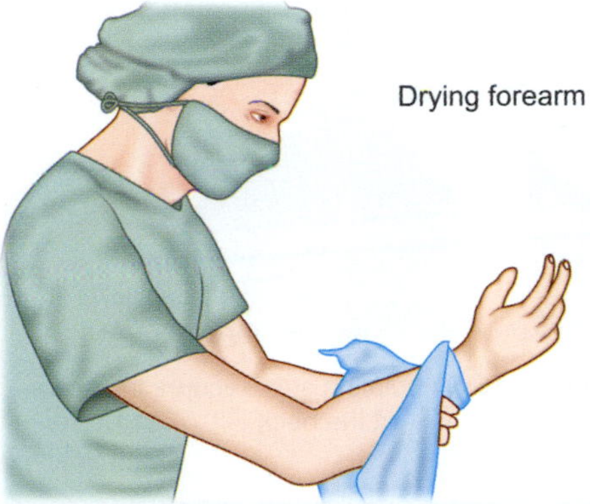

Figure 1.9: Drying hands using rotating movements

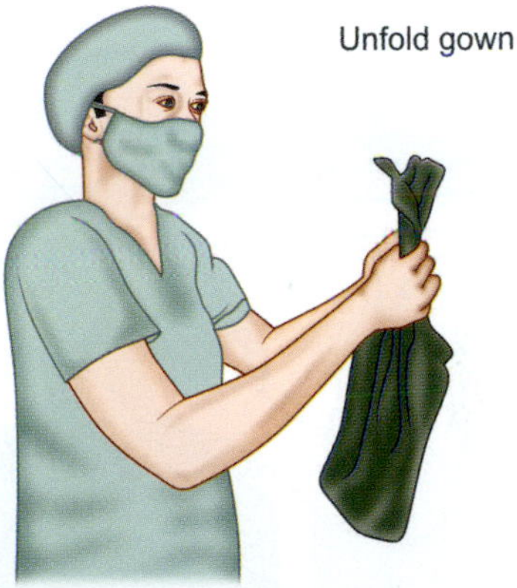

Unfold gown

Figure 1.12: Unfold the gown

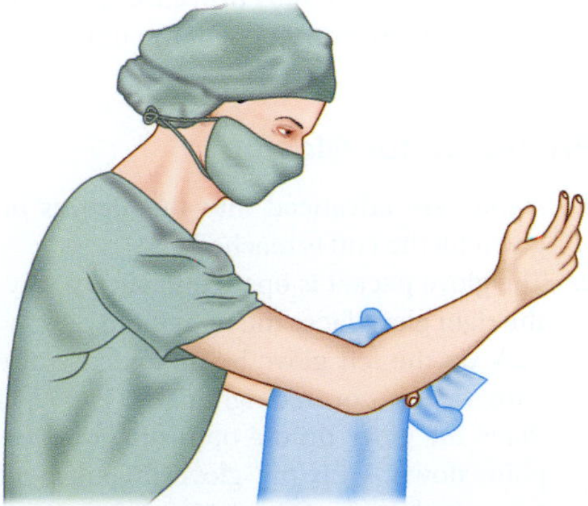

Figure 1.10: Drying the forearms

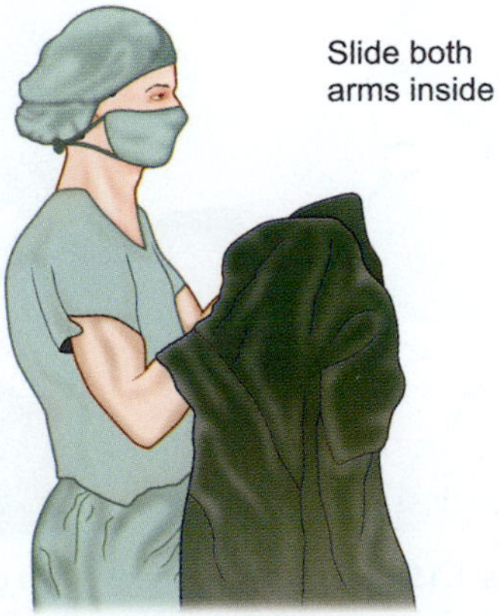

Slide both
arms inside

Figure 1.13: Slide hands and arms into the sleeves

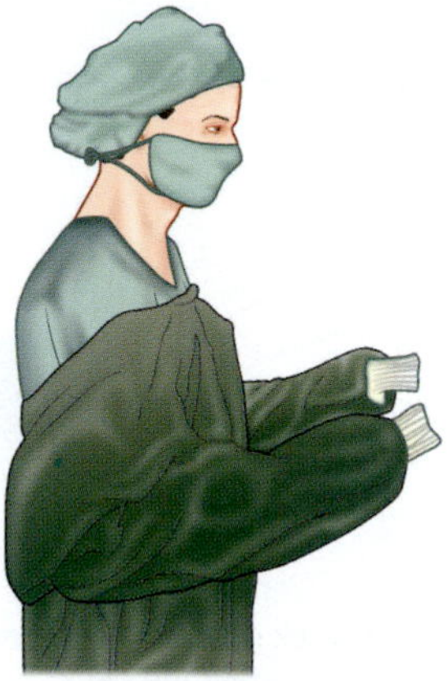

Figure 1.14: Slide the arms into the sleeves completely but without protruding fingers out of cuffs

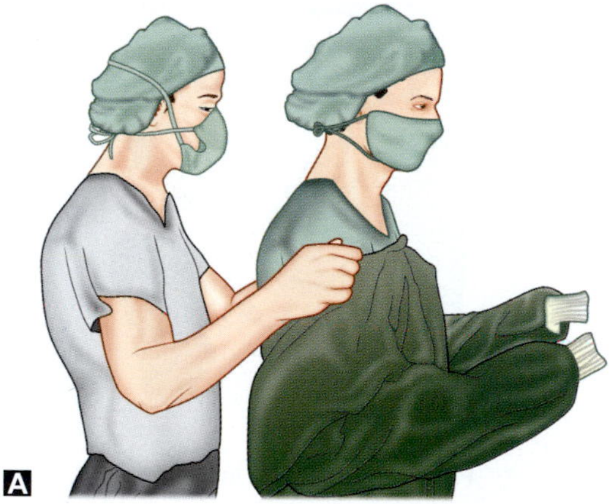

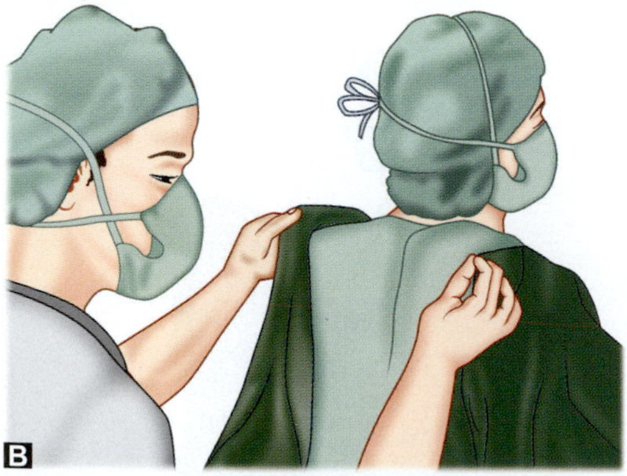

Figures 1.15A and B: Adjustment of the gown over the shoulder

the gown. The gown is secured at the back by the circulating staff (Figs 1.15 and 1.16).

Rules to observe while wearing sterile gowns and gloves:

1. Do not drop your hands below the level of the umbilicus or below the sterile working area.
2. Never place hands behind the back.
3. Gloved hands must be kept within full view at all times.
4. Do not tuck gloved hands under the arm pits, as axillary region is considered contaminated.
5. Never touch an un-sterile area with gloved hands.

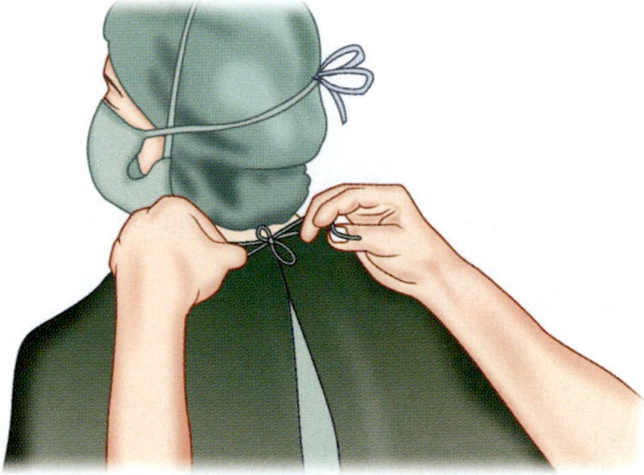

Figure 1.16: Circulating staff secures the gown at the neck

SURGICAL GLOVING TECHNIQUE

Closed gloving is the technique of choice because gloves are handled through the fabric of the gown sleeves, thereby preventing bare hands from coming into contact with the outside of the glove.

Procedure for Gloving

1. Hands are advanced into the sleeves of the gown till the cuff is reached.
2. The glove packet is opened in such a way that the right glove faces the right hand.
3. Pick up the left glove by its folded cuff edge with a sleeve covered right hand (Fig. 1.17).
4. Place the glove on the opposite gown sleeve, palm down, with the glove fingers pointing towards shoulder (Figs 1.18 to 1.20). The palm

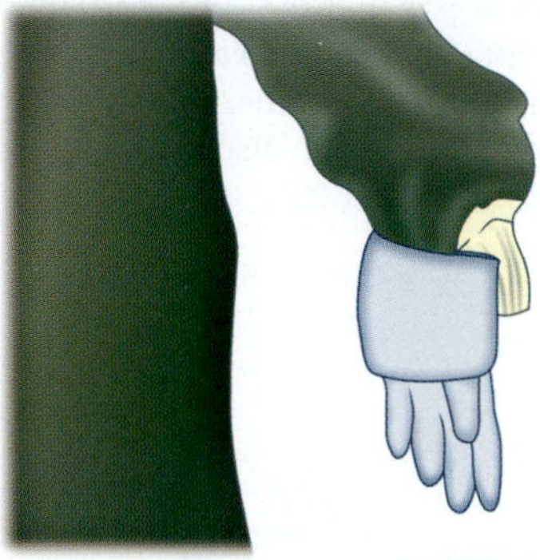

Figure 1.17: Picking up a glove by its folded cuff edge with a sleeve-covered hand

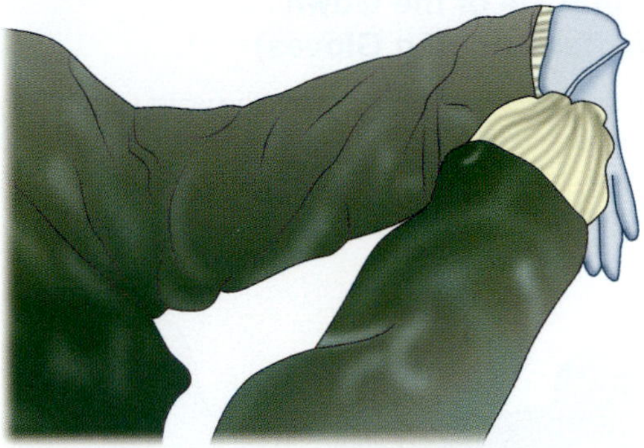

Figure 1.20: Glove should be placed in such a way that the rolled edge of the gloved cuff is at the junction of gown cuff and sleeve

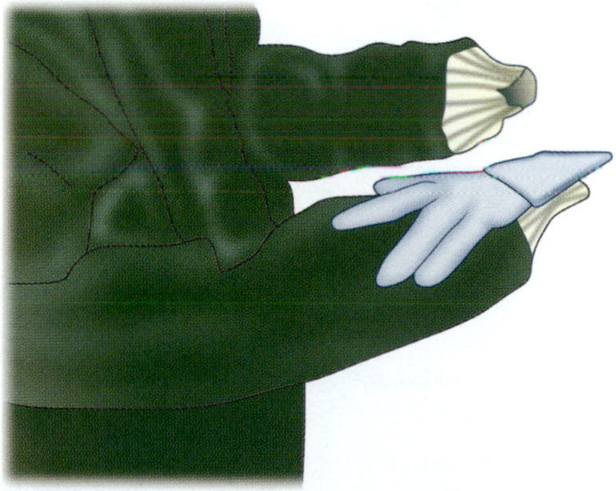

Figure 1.18: Place the glove on the opposite sleeve

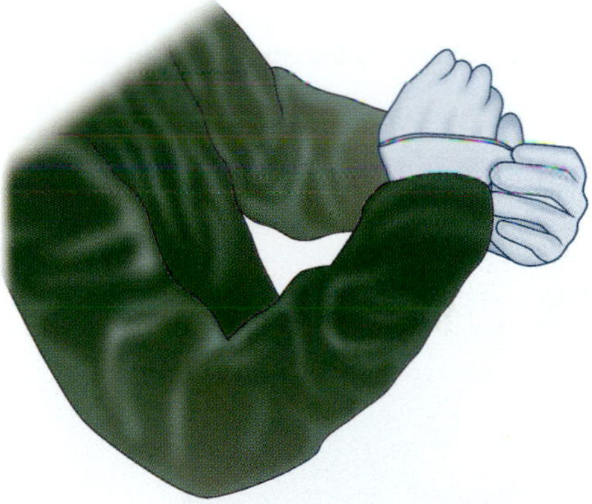

Figure 1.21: Hold the bottom rolled edge of the glove with thumb and index finger

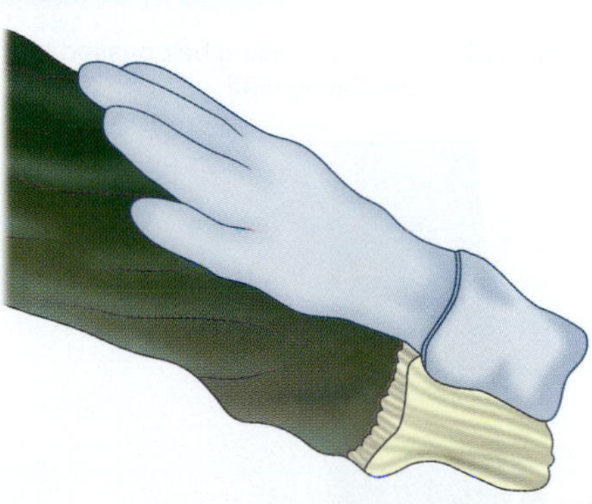

Figure 1.19: Place the glove on the opposite sleeve (Left glove on right sleeve)

of the hand inside the gown sleeve must be facing upwards towards the palm of the glove. Hold the bottom rolled edge of the glove with thumb and index finger (Fig. 1.21).

5. Grasp the uppermost edge of the glove's cuff with the opposite hand and stretch the cuff of the glove over the hand. Put left hand covered with gown sleeve into glove's cuff (Fig. 1.22). Advance your fingers out of the gown sleeve into the cuff of the glove and adjust them into the respective finger stalk. Adjust the glove over the gown sleeve with the right hand covered with gown sleeve (Fig. 1.23).
6. Don the right glove in a similar manner.

Final Tie of the Gown (After Donning Gloves)

If the gown is made of cotton, the waist tie can only be passed around and behind the gowned person by a scrubbed and gowned member of staff, to maintain sterility.

If the gown is a paper disposable one, then a disposable tab attached to the waist tie can be handed to a nonscrubbed member of staff to be passed around the waist. The disposable tab is then discarded (Figs 1.24 to 1.28).

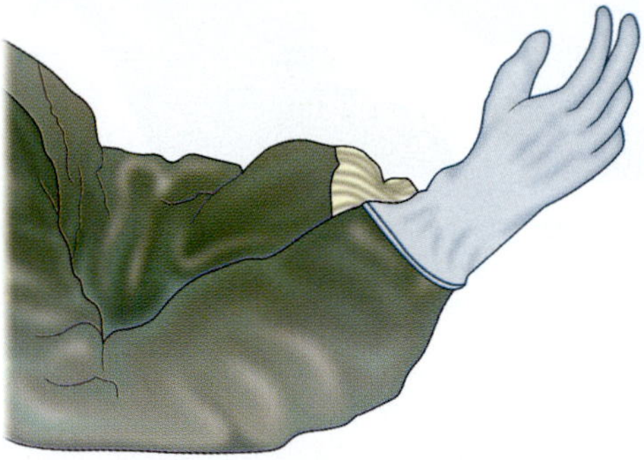

Figure 1.22: Stretching the glove cuff over the hand

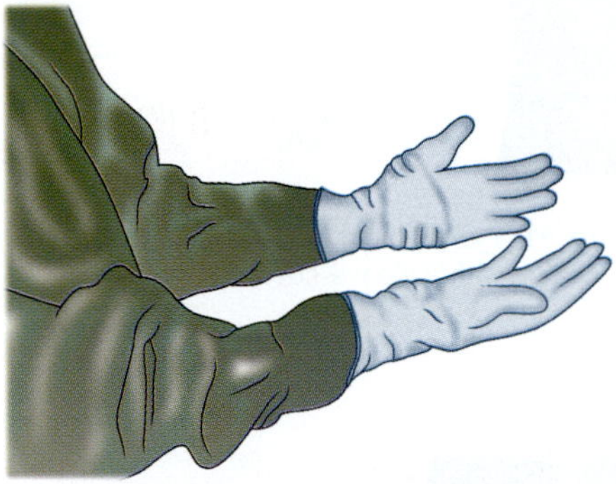

Figure 1.23: Pulling the glove on to the hand

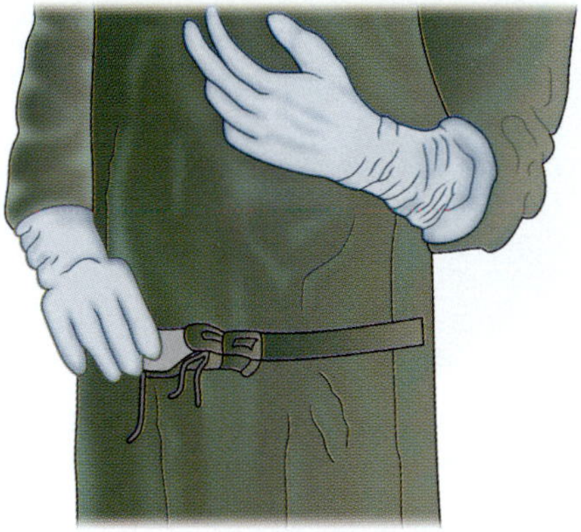

Figure 1.24: Scrubbed person holds the paper tab attached to the belt and belt tie

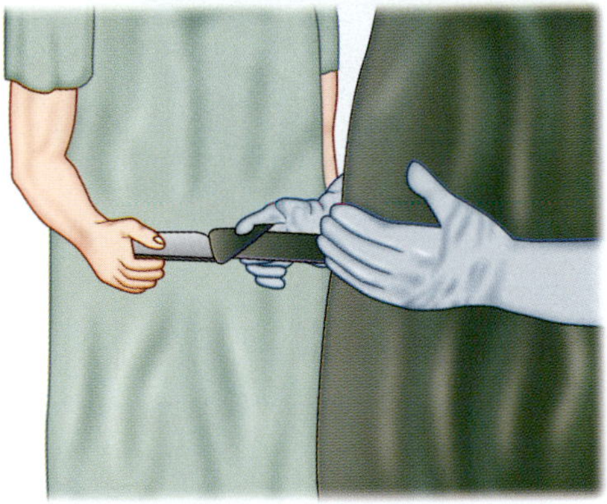

Figure 1.25: Paper tab holding belt passed to circulating staff

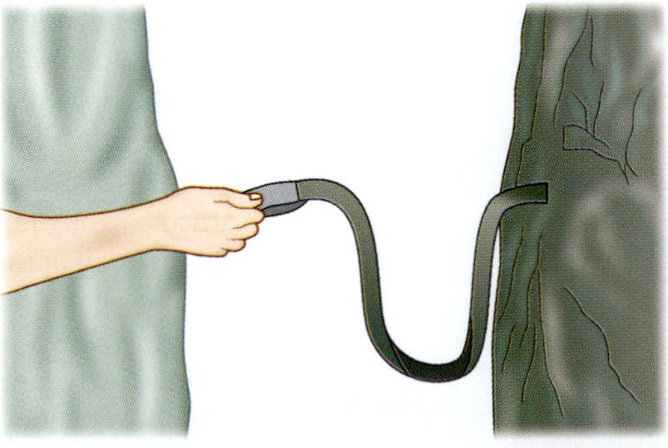

Figure 1.26: Circulating staff holding paper tab comes to the other side of the scrubbed person

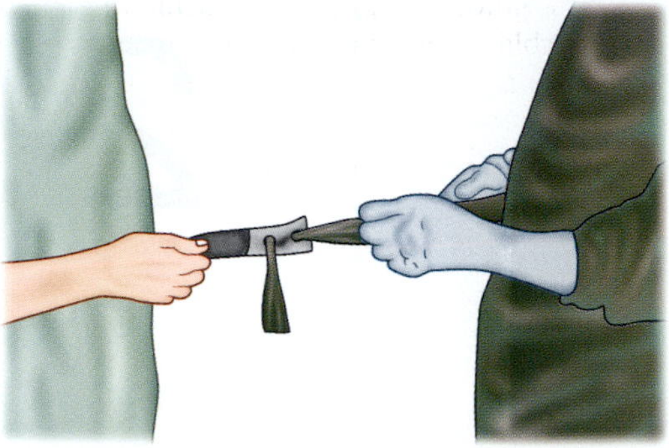

Figure 1.27: Scrubbed person should hold the belt without touching the paper tab and pull out the belt

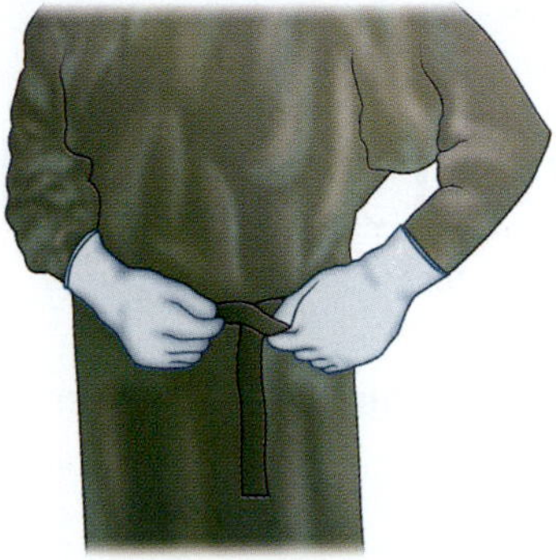

Figure 1.28: Scrubbed person will take hold of the belt tie and tie the belt to it

Key Points

1. The purpose of scrubbing is to reduce the number of organisms on the skin so that the risk to the patient is less if gloves are accidentally perforated during surgery.
2. One can scrub with an antiseptic solution or soap.
3. Recommended scrubbing time is 2 minutes with antiseptic solution and 5 minutes with soap.
4. Scrubbing time does not include rinsing time.
5. While wearing a gown one should touch only the inside or back of the gown.
6. A gown is contaminated if one touches outside of the gown.
7. Closed gloving technique is better than open gloving technique.

Knot Tying Techniques

2

Sudhir Kumar Jain, David L Stoker

The art of knot tying has been developed by man kind ever since the dawn of civilisation. As is evident from historical accounts, ancient cultures had accomplished rope makers in the population who realised that rope cannot serve any useful purpose unless tied by secure knots. And so it appears that man learnt the art of rope making and knot tying at around the same time. Knotted ropes have played an important role in human history from construction of homes to creation of bridges and notably in shipping. Knots have religious and symbolic connotations across cultures. An example being the Hindu marriage ceremony where the physical act of tying parts of the couple's clothing together is a metaphor for the union of two souls for life.

Knots are used in surgery for the approximation of tissues or for ligation of blood vessels. More than 1400 knots have been described in the Encyclopedia on knots, but only a few are used in performing surgeries. The type of surgical knot used depends upon the suture material, location, depth of the incision and the amount of stress placed upon the wound. Multifilament sutures are easier to tie than monofilament sutures, because they have a high coefficient of friction and the knots remain in same position as they are laid down. In contrast knots tied with the monofilament sutures have a tendency to loosen because of a low coefficient of friction. Monofilament sutures have memory, and they tend to return to their original resting shape. While tying knots, surgeons must work slowly and meticulously, as undue speed in knot tying may result in a poor tie, slippage and possible undesirable consequences.

SAFE PRINCIPLES OF KNOT TYING

1. The completed knot must be firm to avoid slipping.
2. Knot must be as small as possible and ends should be cut short.
3. While tying a knot, friction between strands must be avoided as this can weaken the suture.
4. Avoid excessive tension on the suture while applying the knot.
5. Tension on the final throw should be as nearly horizontal as possible.
6. Care should be taken not to damage the suture material when handling it, e.g. crushing of the suture material between the jaws of a hemostat.
7. Tension should be maintained on the knot after the first loop has been tied to avoid loosening of the throw.
8. Extra ties do not add to the strength of a properly tied and squared knot but only add to the bulk.

METHODS OF KNOT TYING

1. Hand tied knot
2. Instrument tied knot
3. Endoscopically tied knot.

A Hand Tied Knot can be

1. Granny knot
2. Square knot or reef knot
3. Surgeon's knot
4. Reverse surgeon's knot
5. Double-double knot.

A hand tied knot can be created either by one or both hands.

IMPORTANCE OF KNOT TYING

The knot is the weakest link in a tied surgical suture. The consequences of suboptimal and faulty knot construction may be disastrous. For example, massive haemorrhage may result from a poorly tied knot on a large artery. Knot disruption may also lead to abdominal wound dehiscence or an incisional hernia. It is important to understand the mechanical performance of a united and knotted suture, as an important complication in a suture's mechanical performance includes knot breakage and knot slippage.

COMPONENTS OF A KNOTTED SUTURE LOOP

A Tied Suture has Three Components

1. The loop created by a knot maintains approximation of the divided wound edge.
2. A knot is composed of a number of throws snagged against each other. A throw is a wrapping or weaving of two strands.
3. Ears or the cut ends ensure that the loop will not become untied because of knot slippage.

Each throw within a knot can be either a single or double throw. A single throw is formed by wrapping the two strands around each other so that the rotation of the wrap is 360°. In a double throw, the free end of the strand is passed twice instead of once around the other strand. The rotation of this double wrap throw is 720°.

Square knot: When the right ear and the loop of the two throws exit on the same side of the knot or parallel to each other.

Granny knot: When the right ear and loop exit or cross different sides of the knot.

Surgeon's knot: It is comprised of an initial double throw followed by a single throw.

Reverse surgeon's knot: It is comprised of an initial double throw followed by a single throw and subsequently a double-wrap throw.

Double-double knot: It consists of two double throws.

One handed square knot technique: It can be tied using either hand.

This type of knot is employed if using a suture with a needle attached to it. After passing the needle through the tissue, the thread is pulled until the end of the suture attached to the needle is long. One handed tying of a knot uses two types of throws, i.e. index finger throw and middle finger throw. If the short end is away from the operator then the index finger throw is used. If the short end is towards the operator, the middle finger throw is used. If the short end is towards the right hand side of operator, then one can use either index finger throw by left hand or middle finger throw by right hand. If the short end is towards the left side of operator, then one can use middle finger by left hand or index finger throw by right hand.

Crossing of hands at the end of each throw is of paramount importance. It means that if the short end is away from the operator, it should come towards the operator at the end of the throw. Crossing of hands is also known as "squaring the knot" and ensures that the knot does not become an unsafe slip knot.

Steps

1. Hold the short end of suture between the thumb and ring finger of the left hand with the loop over the extended left index finger which has been kept free. Hold the long end of the suture in between the right thumb and right index finger. Abduct the left index finger, so that short end of suture forms a loop over it (Fig. 2.1).
2. Bring the long end of suture held in right hand over loop of short end held in the left hand, by moving the right hand away from you so that it crosses in front of the short end (Fig. 2.2).
3. Bring the index finger of left hand in front of the short end of suture held between left thumb and ring finger (Fig. 2.3).
4. Pronate the left hand so that the left index finger brings the thread held between left thumb and ring finger inside the loop.
5. Pull the thread out of loop by grasping it between the left index and middle finger and

complete the throw by bringing the left hand towards you and the right hand away from you (Fig. 2.4).

6. Continue to hold the short end of the suture in the left hand between the thumb and index finger. Flex and abduct the left index finger so that it lies at a right angle to the remaining left hand fingers (Fig. 2.5).
7. Bring the thread held in the right hand across the left middle finger towards the operator to cross the left handed thread (Fig. 2.6).
8. Use middle finger of left hand to bring the short end under the right handed strand of suture (Figs 2.7 to 2.11).

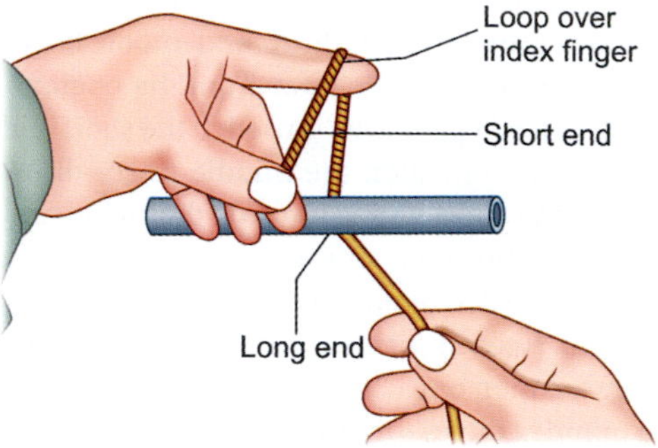

Figure 2.1

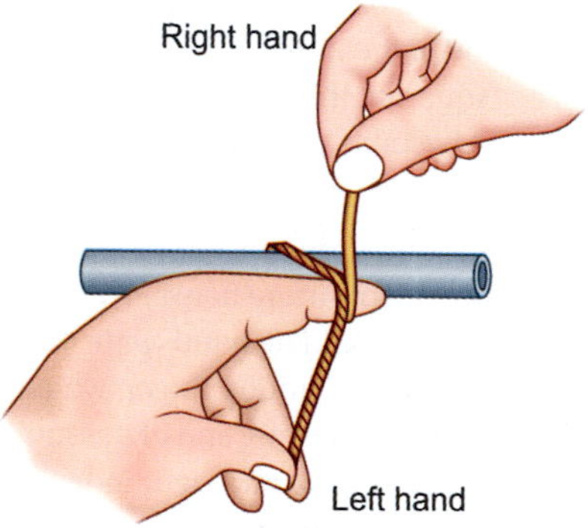

Figure 2.2

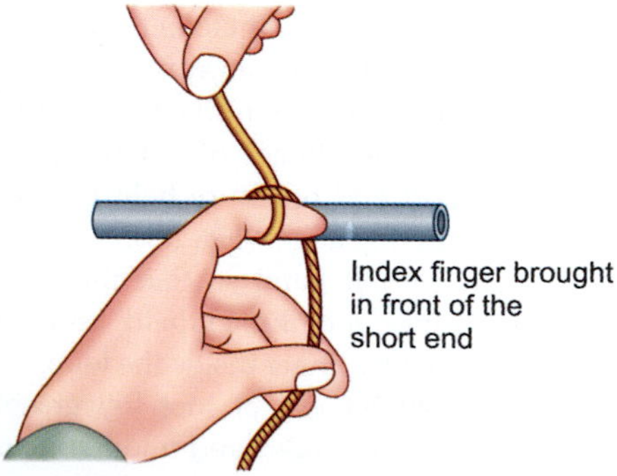

Figure 2.3

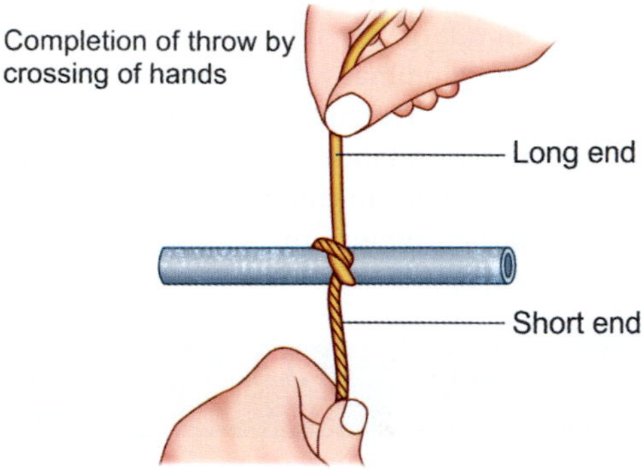

Figure 2.4

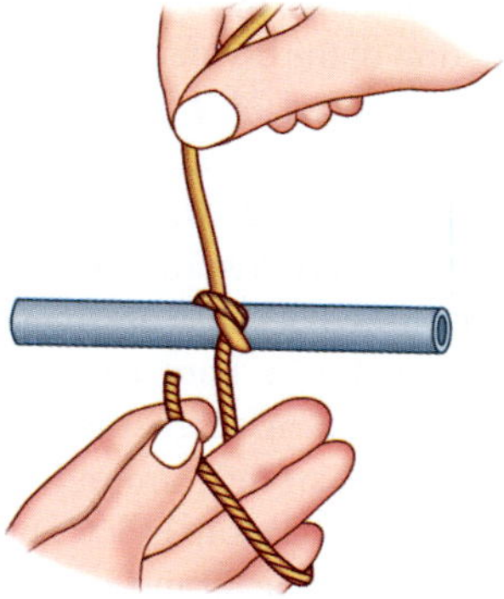

Figure 2.5

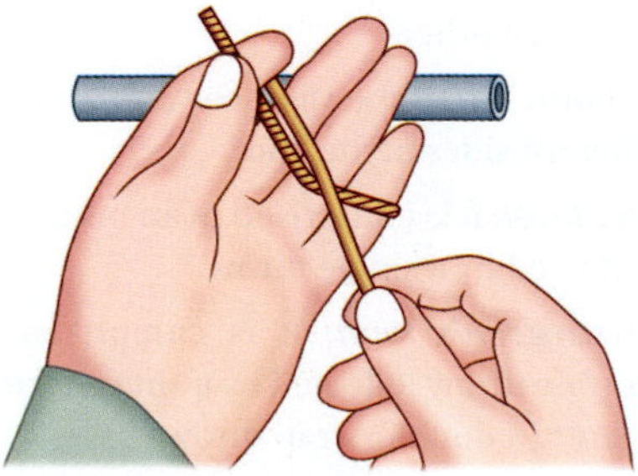

Figure 2.6

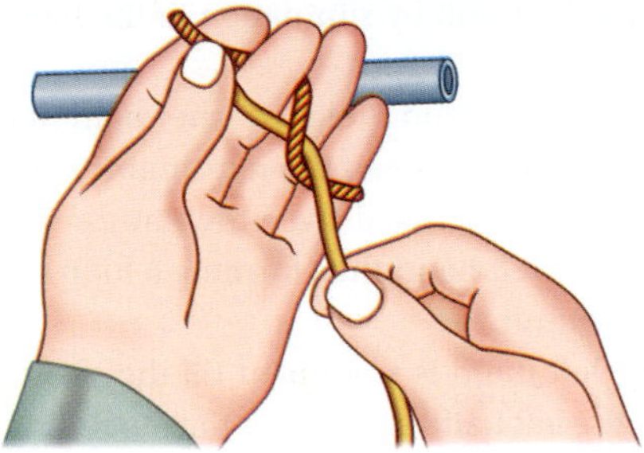

Figure 2.7

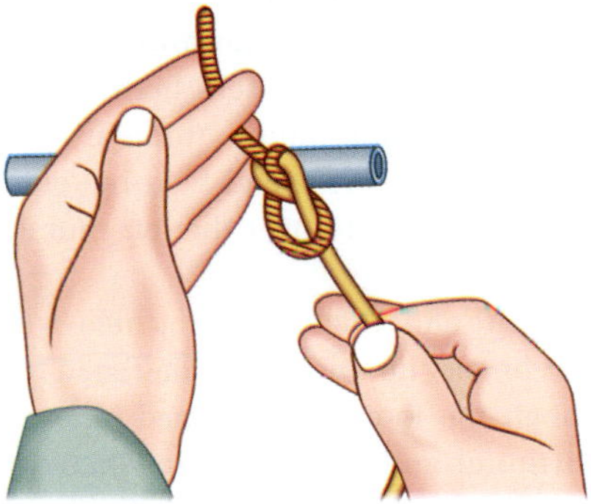

Figure 2.8

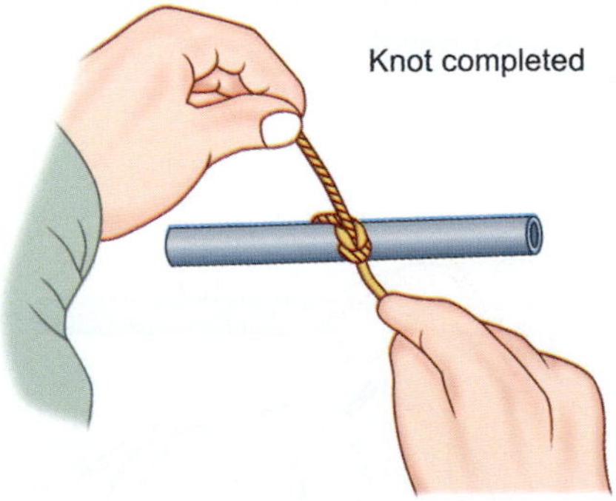

Figure 2.9

Figures 2.1 to 2.9: Various steps of single handed reef knot

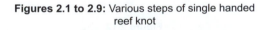

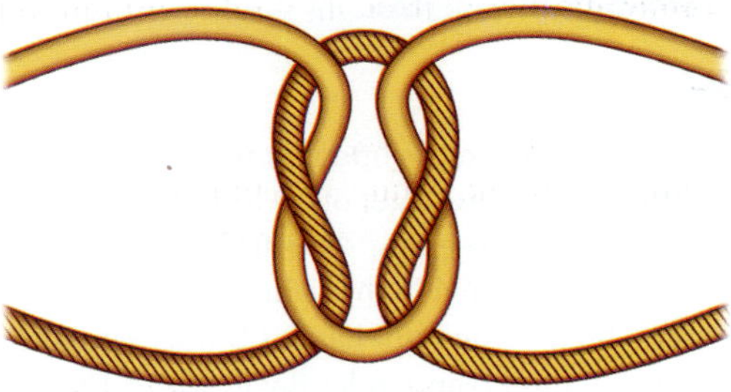

Figure 2.10A: Cross-section of completed reef knot

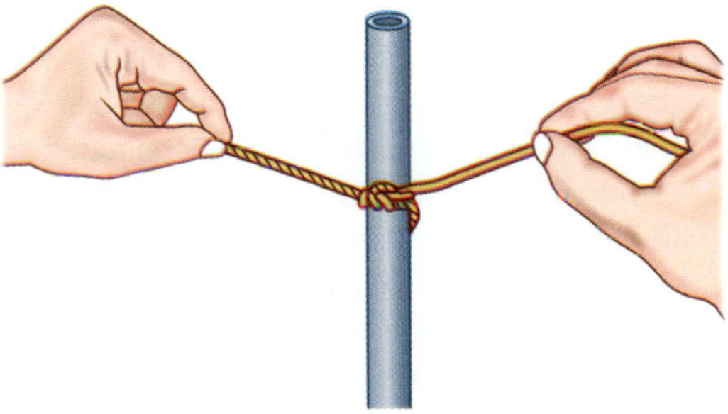

Figure 2.10B: Completed reef knot final appearance

9. Grasp the short end between the left middle and ring finger and bring the short end away from you and tighten the knot.

Single Handed Surgeon's Knot

In this knot a double throw is performed in the first half knot. To create this knot the short end is drawn twice through the loop made over the index finger before pulling the short end towards the operator. Knot is completed by making a middle finger throw.

Double Handed Reef Knot

A double handed reef knot is used if there is a free suture without the needle attached to it. So instead of the short end and long end, there will be two equal ends. One end away from operator and one end towards the operator.

Steps

1. End away from the operator is placed over the extended index finger of the left hand and held in the palm keeping the left thumb free. The other end is held in the right hand (Fig. 2.11).
2. End held in the right hand is brought between the left thumb and index finger (Fig. 2.12).
3. Left hand is turned inwards by pronation and thumb is brought under the suture held by the left hand to form the first loop (Fig. 2.13).
4. Suture end held in the right hand is crossed over the loop formed on the left thumb and is transferred to be held between thumb and index finger of left hand (Fig. 2.14).
5. The left hand which is still holding the end between index finger and thumb (which was held by right hand initially) is supinated to bring the end held between the left index finger and thumb through the loop formed over the left index finger (Fig. 2.15).
6. The end which is held between the left index finger and thumb is brought through the loop formed over the left index finger, released by the left hand and then grasped by the right hand.
7. First half of the knot is completed by applying horizontal tension and crossing hands (Fig. 2.16).
8. The left index finger is freed from the suture held by the same hand. A loop is formed over the left thumb by supination of the hand (Fig. 2.17).
9. The suture end held by the right hand is brought in between the left thumb and index finger and crossed over the suture which is held by left hand thus forming a loop over the left thumb.
10. The left hand is supinated till the suture held by the left hand slides over the left index finger from left thumb (Fig. 2.18).
11. The suture end held in the right hand is now held between the left thumb and index finger (Fig. 2.19).
12. The left hand is rotated inwards by pronation thus carrying the end held between the left index finger and thumb through the loop formed by the suture end held by remaining fingers of left hand over the left thumb (Fig. 2.20).
13. The suture end which was being held by the left index finger and thumb and has been brought through the loop is re-grasped between the right thumb and index finger and then released by the left index finger and thumb.
14. Second half of the knot is completed by applying horizontal tension across the two ends (Figs 2.20 to 2.22).
15. Final tension on the final throw should be as horizontal as possible.

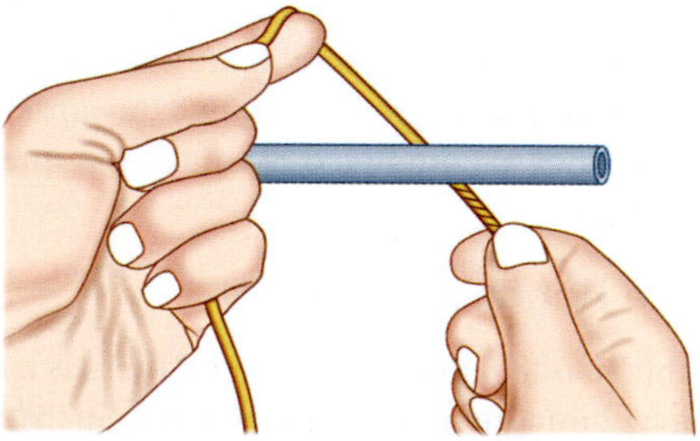

Figure 2.11

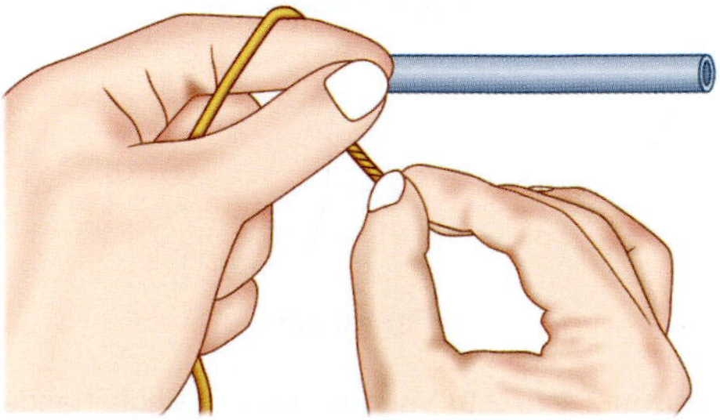

Figure 2.12

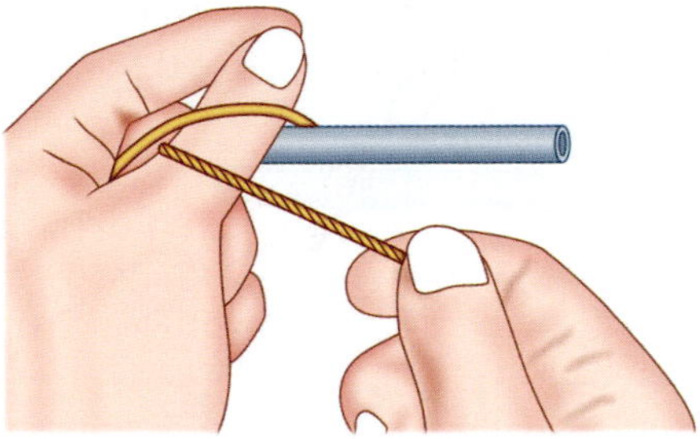

Figure 2.13

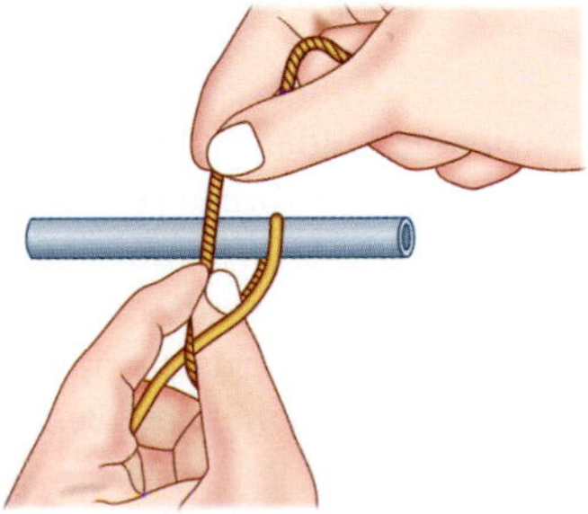

Figure 2.14

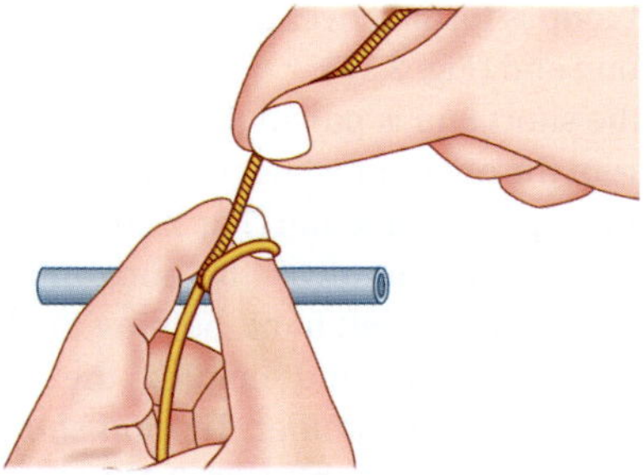

Figure 2.15

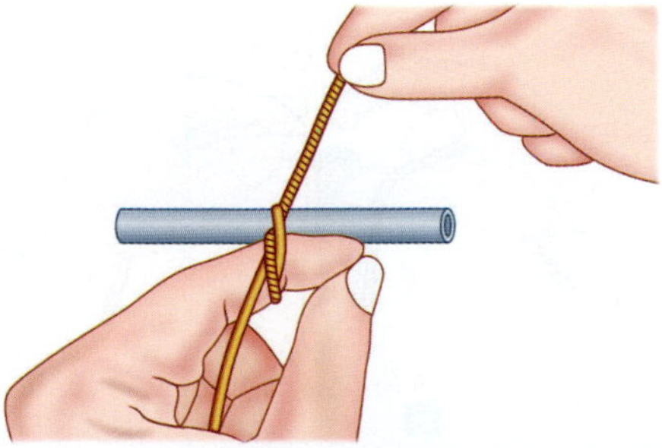

Figure 2.16

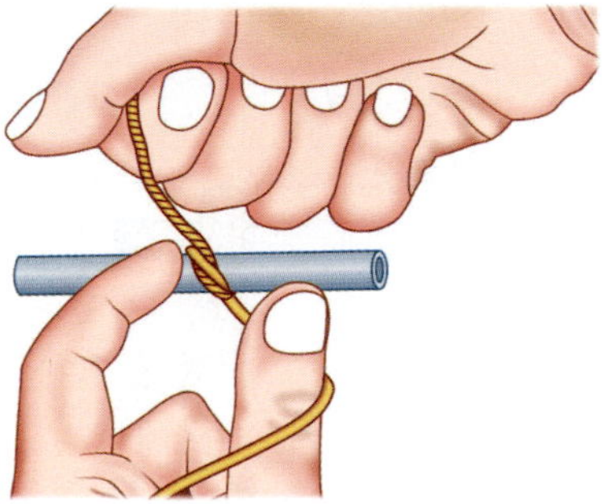

Figure 2.17

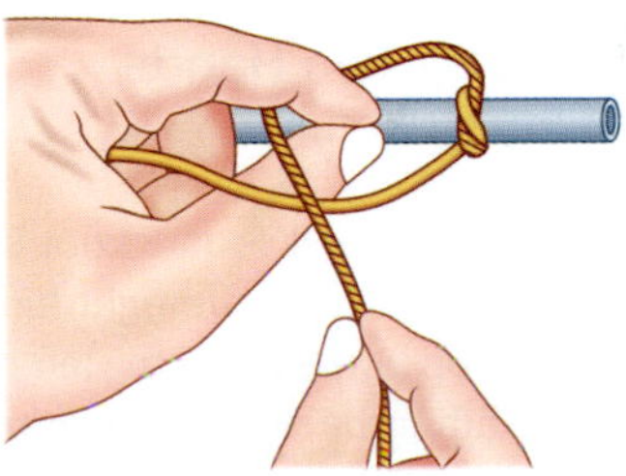

Figure 2.18

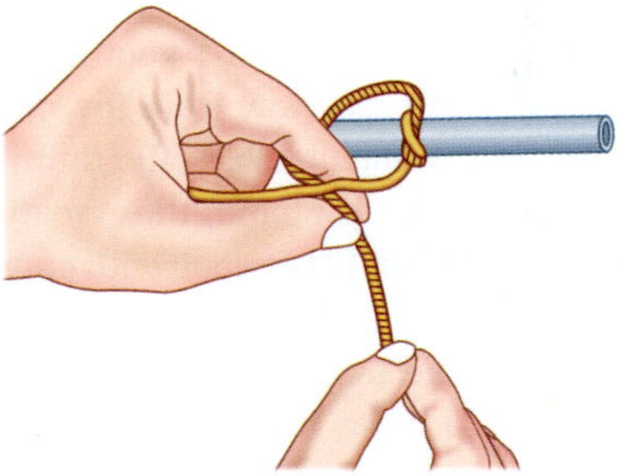

Figure 2.19

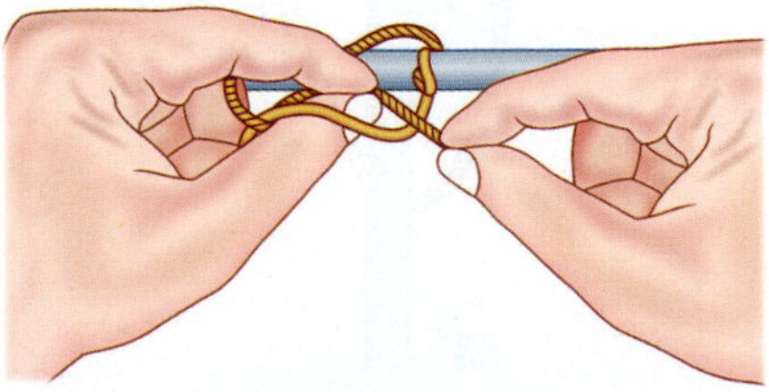

Figure 2.20

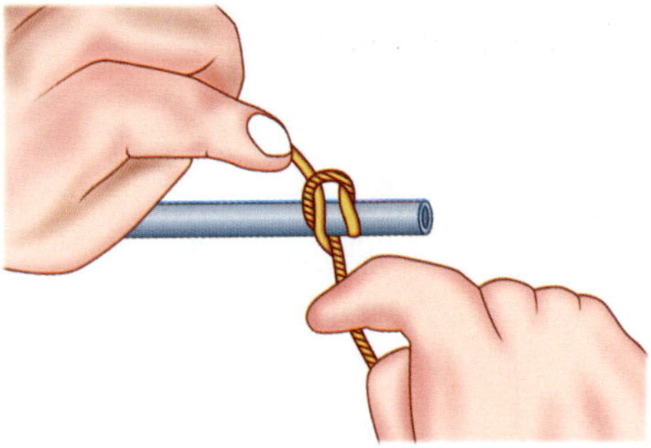

Figure 2.21

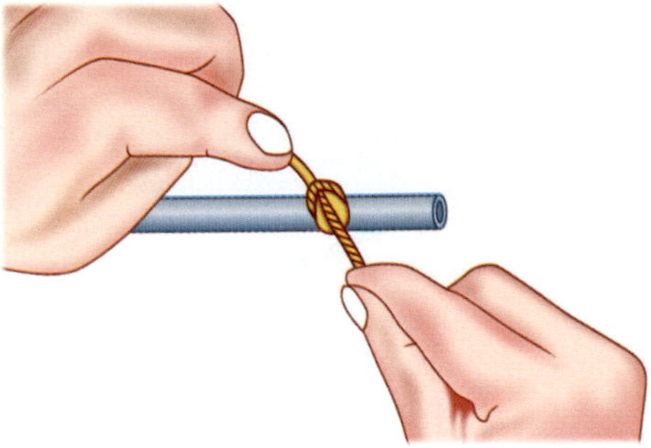

Figure 2.22

Figures 2.11 to 2.22: Various steps of two hand tied reef knot

Surgeon's Knot by Two Hands (Figs 2.23 to 2.33)

This differs from a two handed square knot in the first half. The other end held in the right hand is passed through the loop formed over the left index finger twice before pulling the two ends in opposite directions in a horizontal plane.

Instrument tied knot: Instrument tie is useful when one or both ends of the suture material are short.

Steps of instrument tied surgeon's knot:

1. Short end lies freely, away from the operator and long end is held between the thumb and index finger of the left hand, thus creating an English letter '**V**' or '**C**' between both ends (Fig. 2.34).
2. Place the needle holder inside the 'V' or 'C' and make two loops over the needle holder with the long end (Fig. 2.35).
3. The needle holder in the right hand grasps the short end of the thread (Fig. 2.36).
4. First half of the knot is completed by pulling the needle holder towards oneself thus bringing the short end towards the operator (Fig. 2.37).
5. Long end is again held between left thumb and index finger.
6. The needle holder is held in the right hand and again placed in the '**V**' formed by both ends (Fig. 2.38).
7. A loop is formed over the needle holder by the long end (Fig. 2.39).
8. The short end is pulled through the loop away from the operator while pulling the long end in the opposite direction (Fig. 2.40).
9. The knot is completed by horizontal tension applied by the left hand holding the long end and the right hand holding the short end with the needle holder. Tension should be as horizontal as possible (Fig. 2.41).

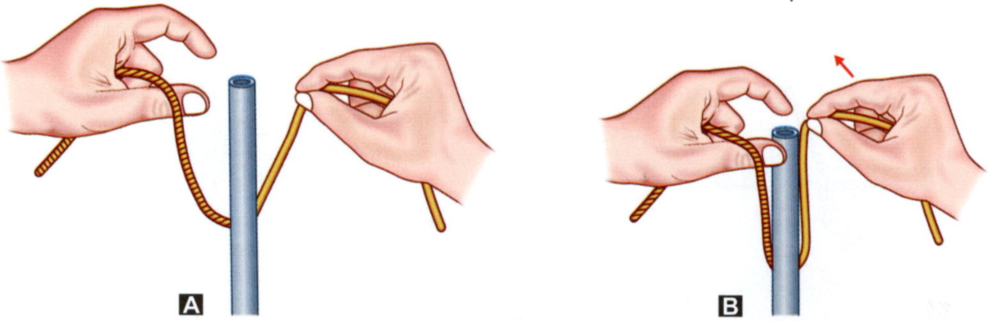

Figures 2.23A and B

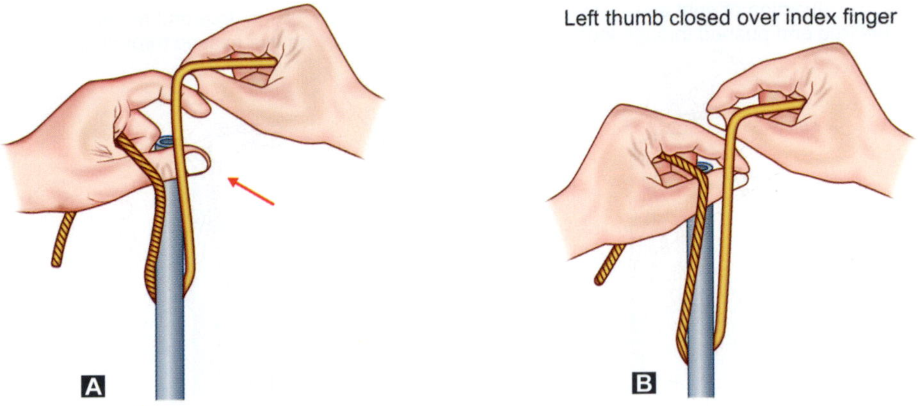

Left thumb closed over index finger

Figures 2.24A and B

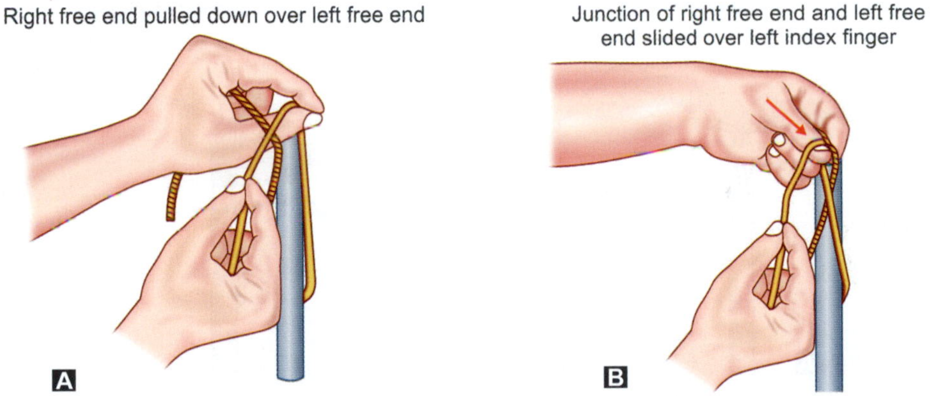

Figures 2.25A and B

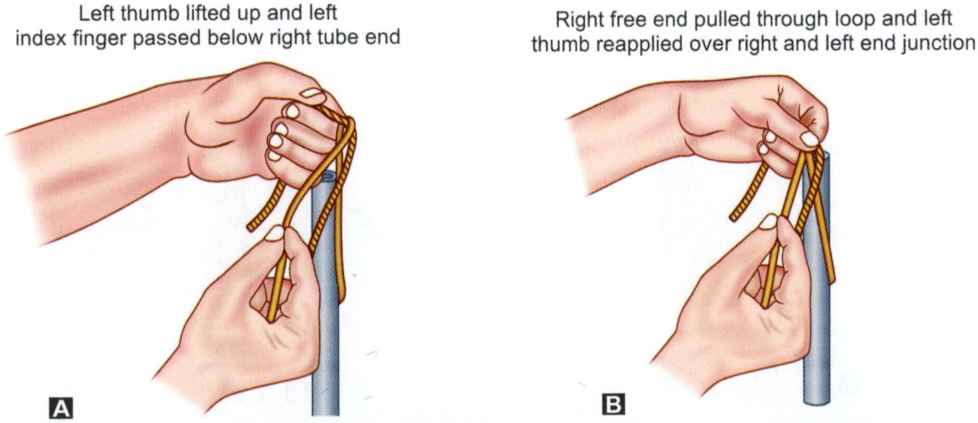

Left thumb lifted up and left index finger passed below right tube end
Right free end pulled through loop and left thumb reapplied over right and left end junction
A
B

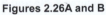

Figures 2.26A and B

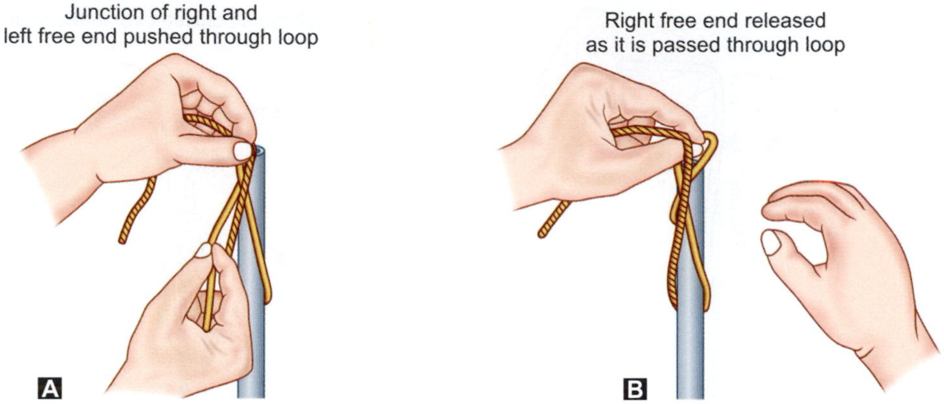

Figures 2.27A and B

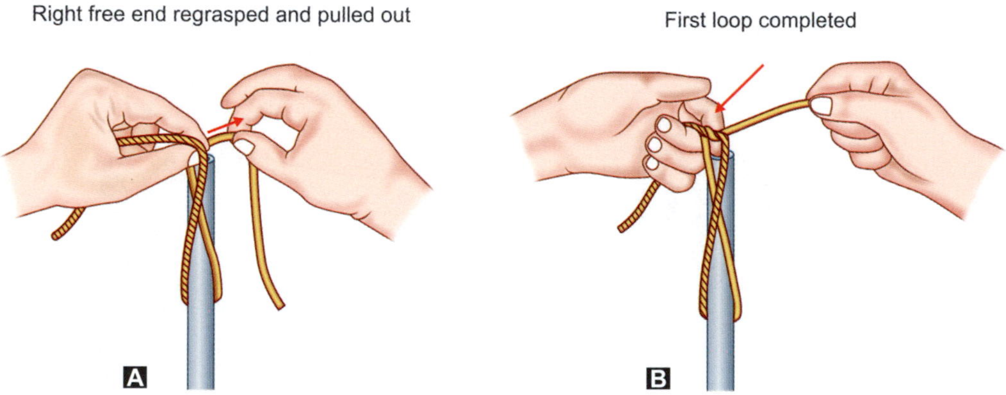

Figures 2.28A and B

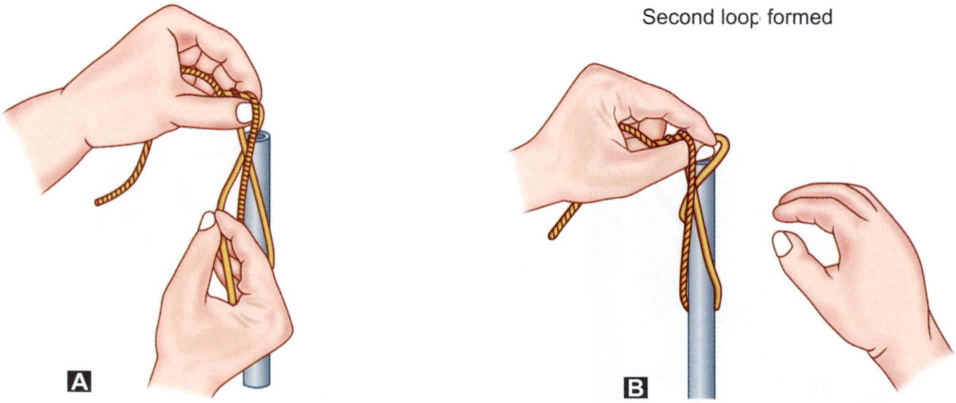

Figures 2.29A and B

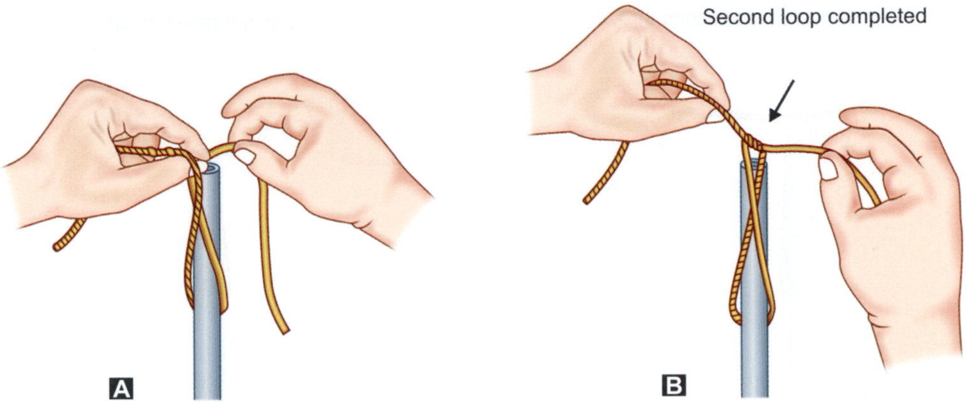

Figures 2.30A and B

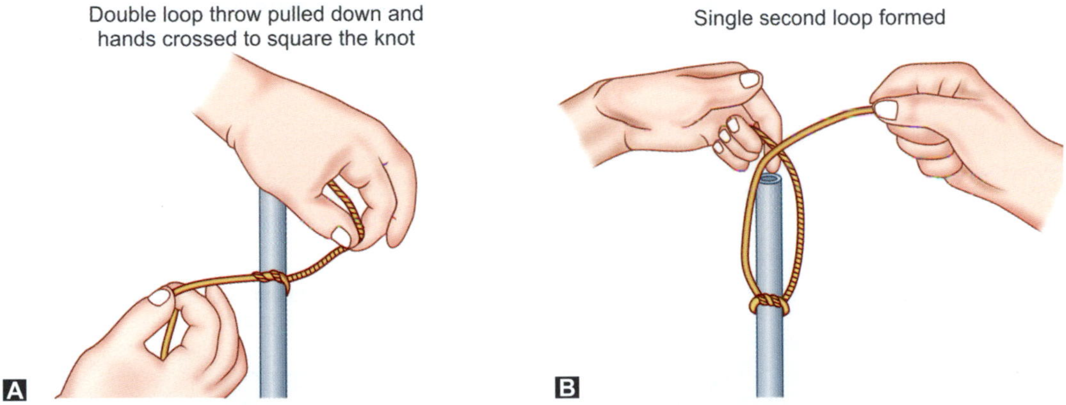

Figures 2.31A and B

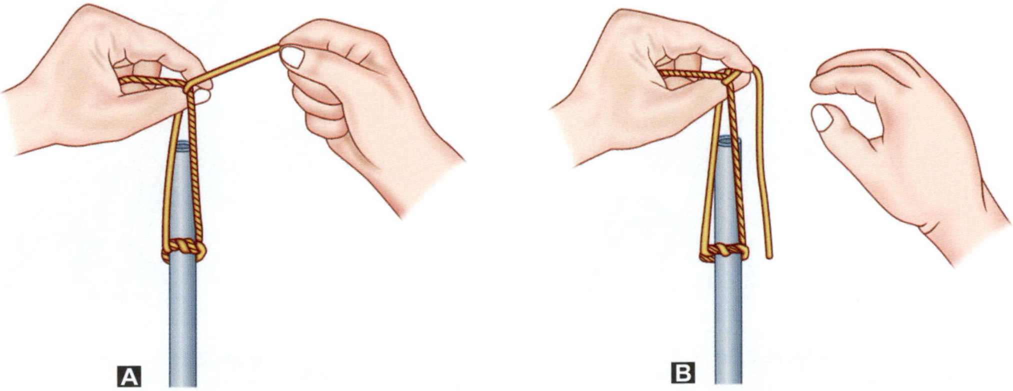

Figures 2.32A and B

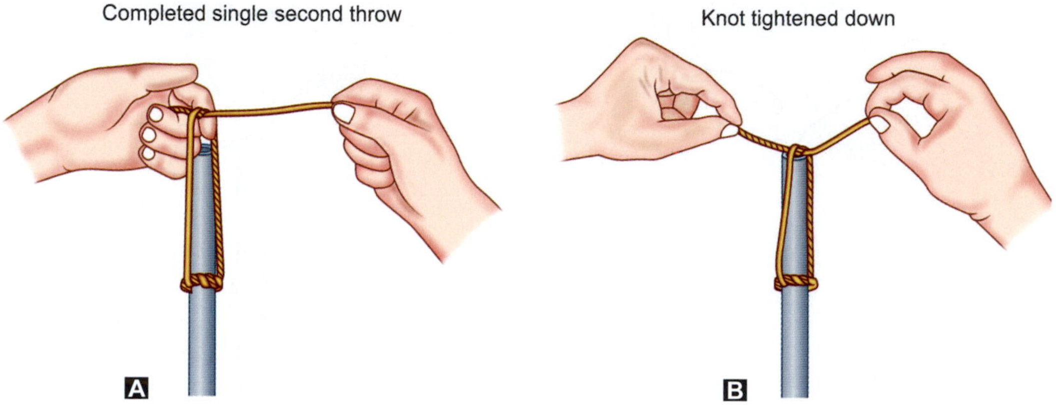

Figures 2.33A and B

Figures 2.23 to 2.33: Various steps of two hand tied surgeon's knot

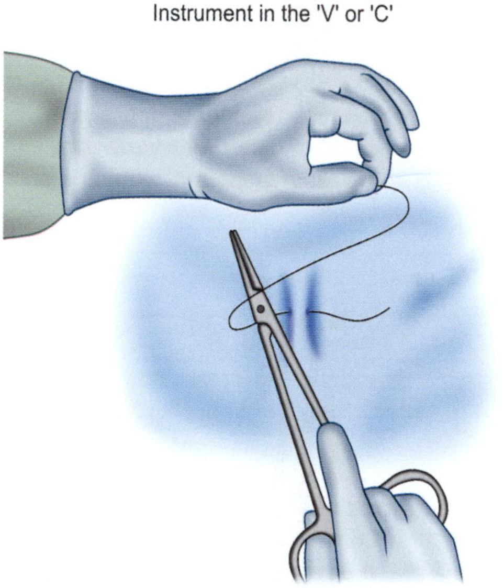

Figure 2.34

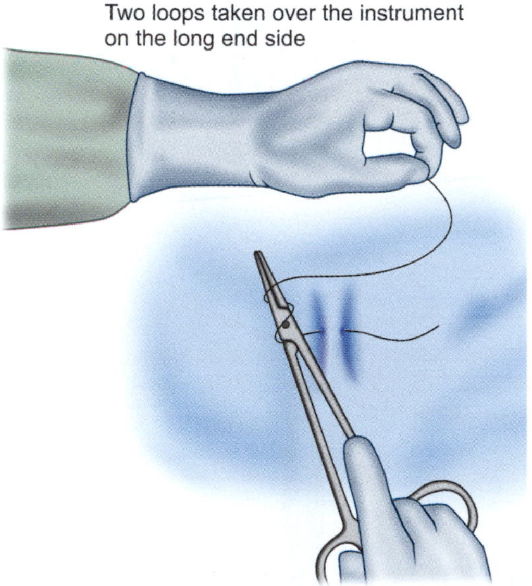

Two loops taken over the instrument
on the long end side

Figure 2.35

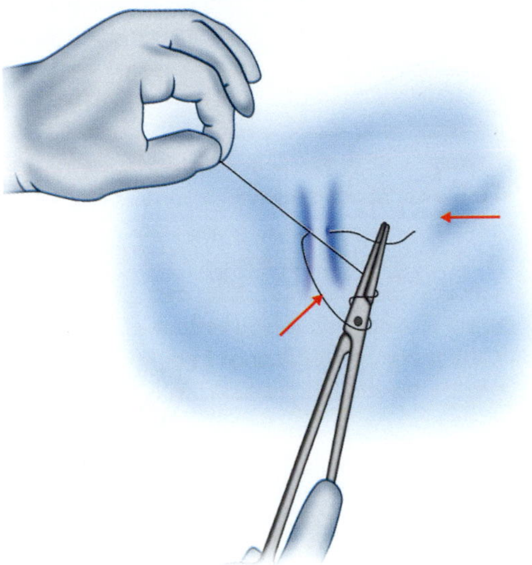

Figure 2.36

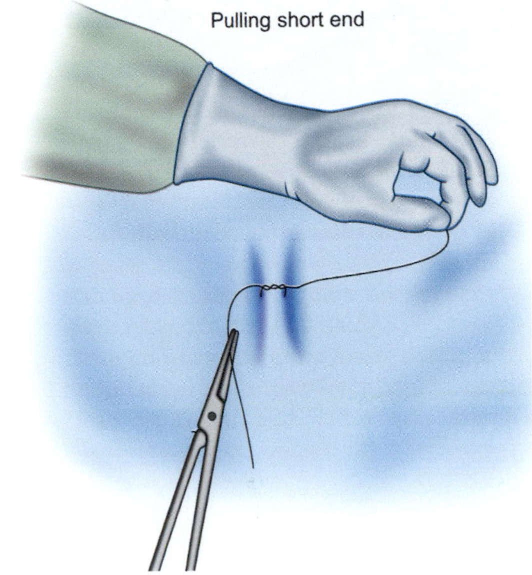

Figure 2.37

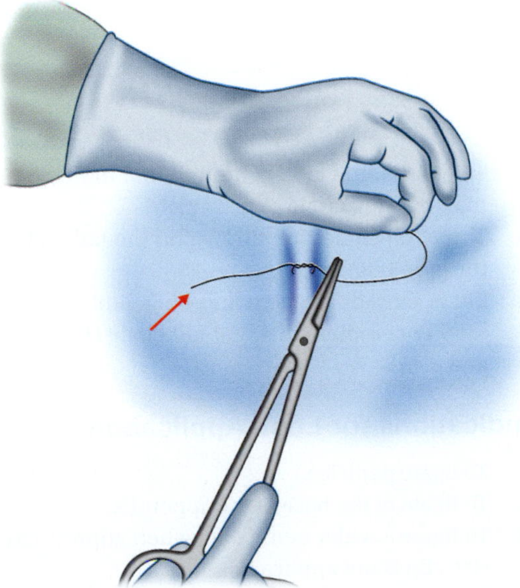

Figure 2.38

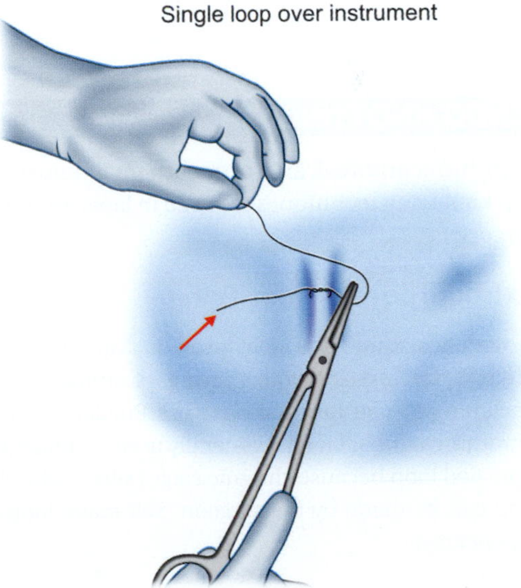

Figure 2.39

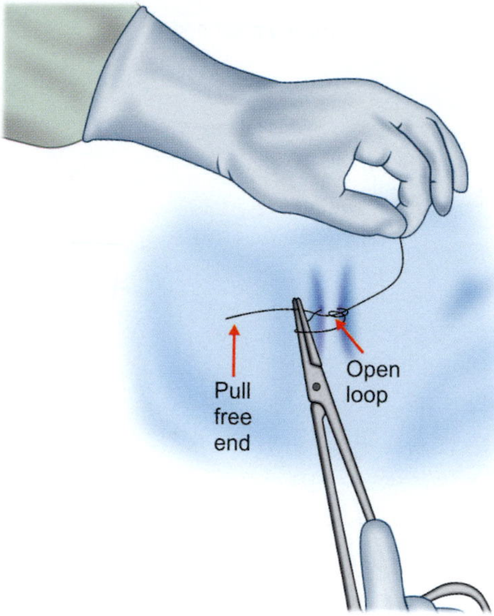

Figure 2.40

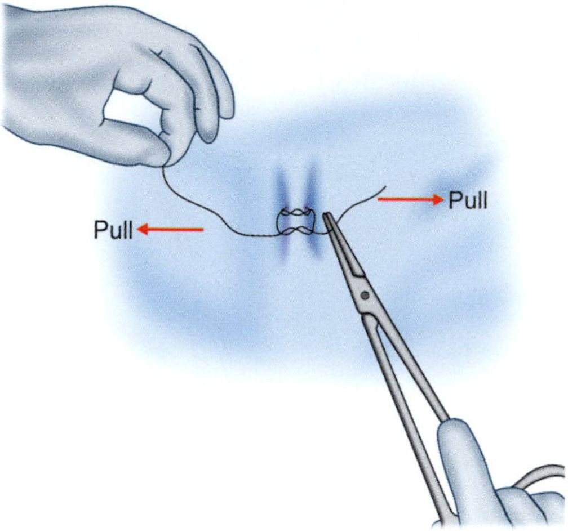

Figure 2.41

Figures 2.34 to 2.41: Various steps of instrument tied surgeon's knot

ENDO KNOTTING

Both intracorporeal and extracorporeal suturing and knot tying techniques are used in laparoscopic surgery.

Extracorporeal Knot Tying

A Roeder's knot is widely used in laparoscopic surgery for extracorporeal tying. Commercially available pre-tied loops also have a Roeder's knot. Chromic catgut or vicryl is generally used for making a pre tied loop because chromic catgut slips easily. A loop can be made by the surgeon. Self-made loops are cheaper.

Steps in Making a Roeder's Knot

1. A loop is formed over the left index finger (Fig. 2.42).
2. Tail end of the loop is brought out of the loop making a full circle (Fig. 2.42).
3. Three full circles are thrown on the tail end of the loop (Fig. 2.43).
4. Tie is closed by encircling both limbs of the loop to complete the final full circle (Figs 2.44 and 2.45).

Indications for Loop Application

1. To ligate pedicles.
2. To ligate of the base of the appendix.
3. To ligate a wider cystic duct when appropriate size clip is not applicable.
4. To control a bleeding vessel which is held by an endograsper.
5. To ligate the hernial sac in an indirect hernia.

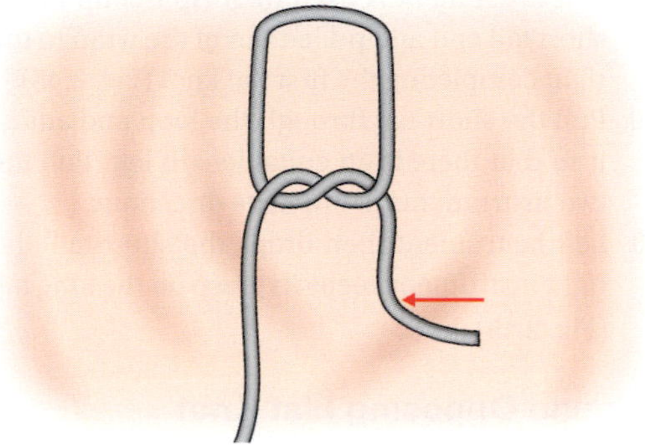

Figure 2.42

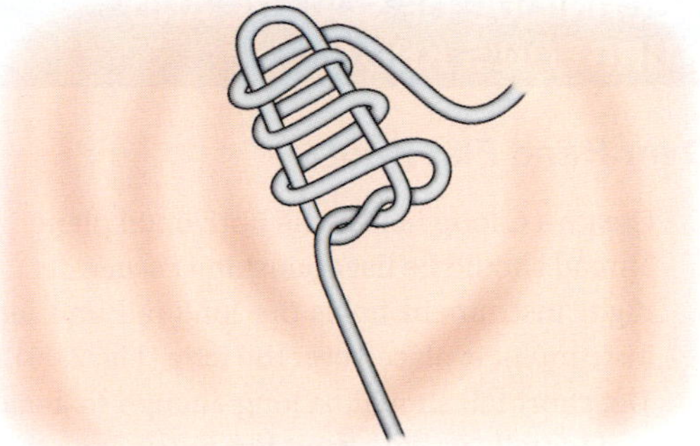

Figure 2.43

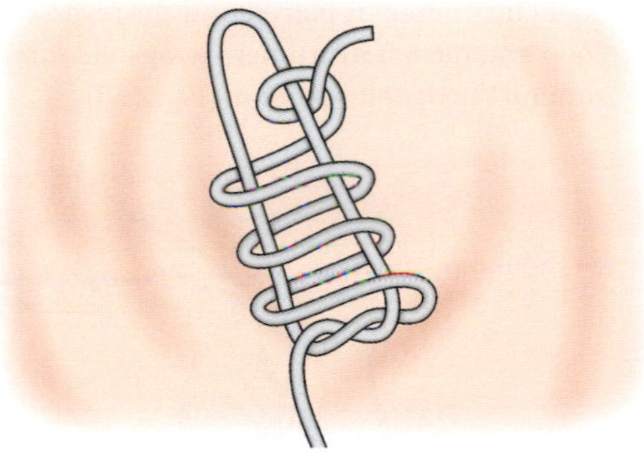

Figure 2.44

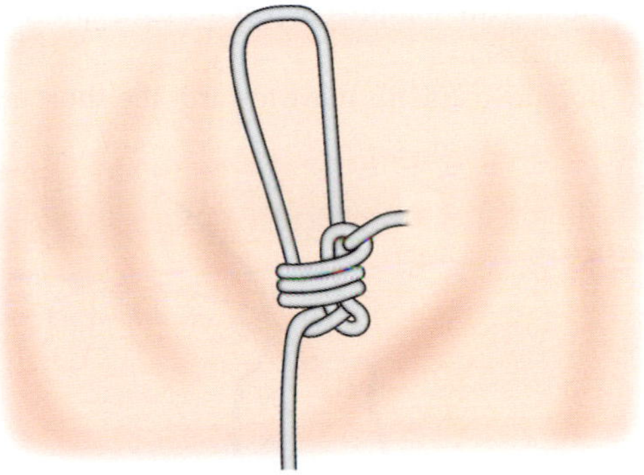

Figure 2.45

Figures 2.42 to 2.45: Various steps of tying Roeder's knot

Intracorporeal Suturing

Prerequisites for making an intracorporeal knot:

1. Suture should be neither too long nor too short. 8–10 cm length of sutures is adequate for one stitch and additional 3 cm for each extra stitch.
2. A curved or "ski" needle is used for endosuturing. Needle is loaded in a reverse way into the reducing sleeve.
3. Left hand forceps should be atraumatic tissue grasping forceps.
4. Needle should be grasped by the needle holder at a right angle to its jaws. Needle tips with high tapering ratio or a "taper cut" tip will penetrate tissue layers more readily.
5. There should be an angle of 60–70° between the right and left hand instrument.
6. Ports should be placed in such a way that principal of triangulation is followed.
7. Vicryl or PDS is ideal for endosuturing.

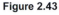

TECHNIQUE OF SQUARE AND SURGEON'S KNOT

Over Hand Flat Knot

1. Create a C loop held in the horizontal plane.
2. Thread should lie flat against the tissue.
3. Right instrument holds the long tail and left instrument is placed over the loop (Fig. 2.46).
4. The short tail should be long enough to avoid accidentally pulling it out but not so long that its end is hidden.
5. Use a large loop to allow sufficient room for movement of both instruments.
6. Use the right instrument to wrap the long tail around the stationary tip of the left instrument (Fig. 2.47).
7. Both instruments move towards the short tail.
8. Left instrument is used to grasp the tip of the short tail end and pulled out of the wrap to the right completing the first flat knot (Fig. 2.48).
9. Pull the short tail through the loop and adjust it so that there is an equal length left. Pull the two instruments in opposite directions.
10. Left instrument then drops the short tail and right instrument keeps its grasp on the long tail (Fig. 2.49).

Second Opposing Flat Knot

1. Right instrument is brought to the left side of the field and rotated clockwise 180°.
2. Right instrument transfers the long tail to the left instrument thus creating a reverse C loop.
3. Right instrument is placed over the reversed C loop and the left instrument wraps the thread around the right instrument (Fig. 2.50).

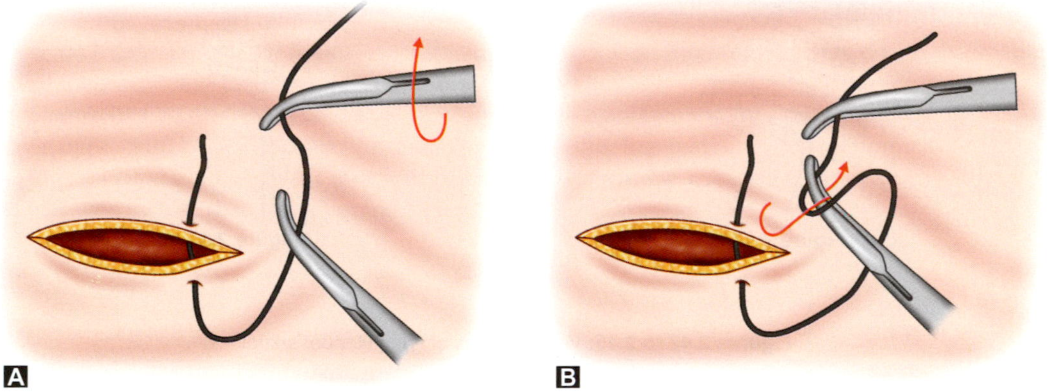

Figures 2.46Aand B

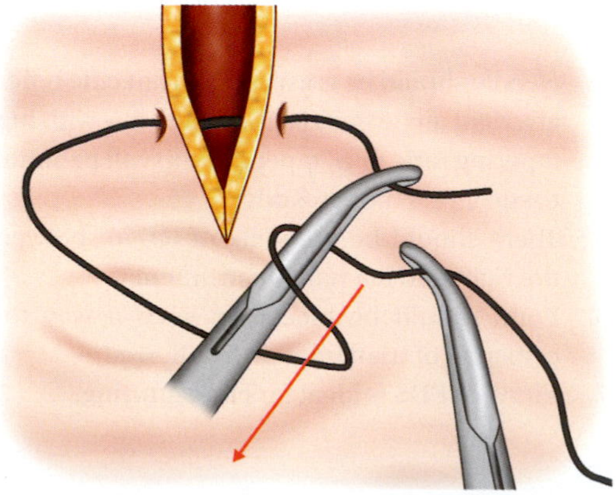

Figure 2.47

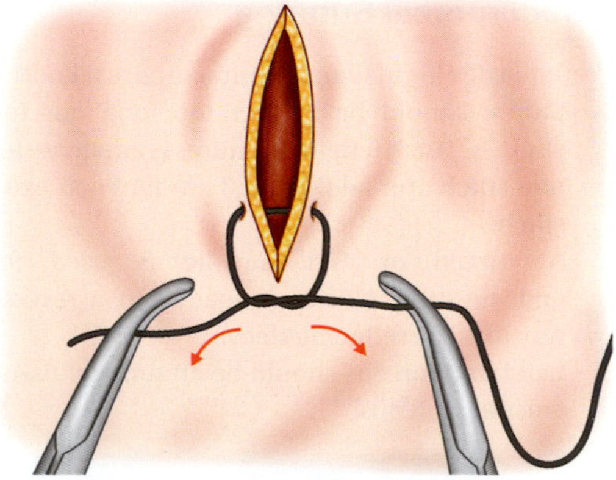

Figure 2.48

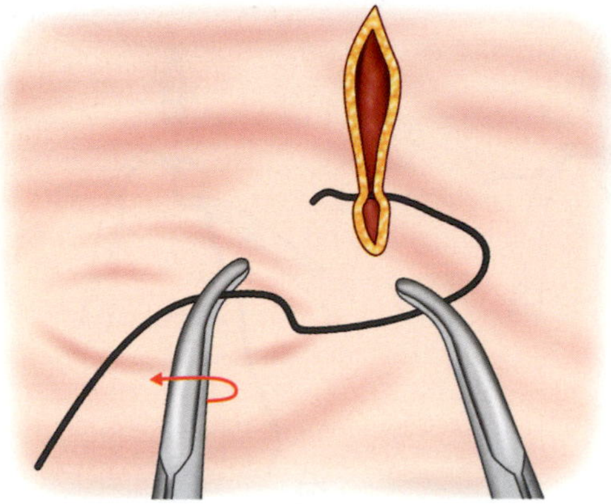

Figure 2.49

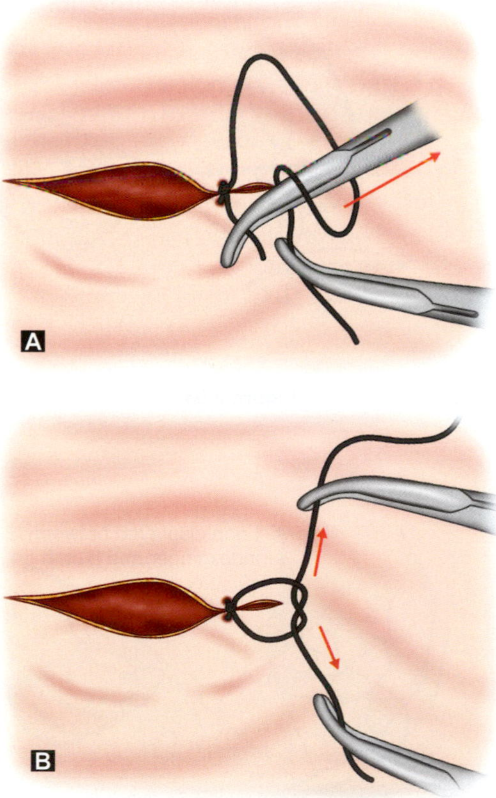

Figures 2.50A and B

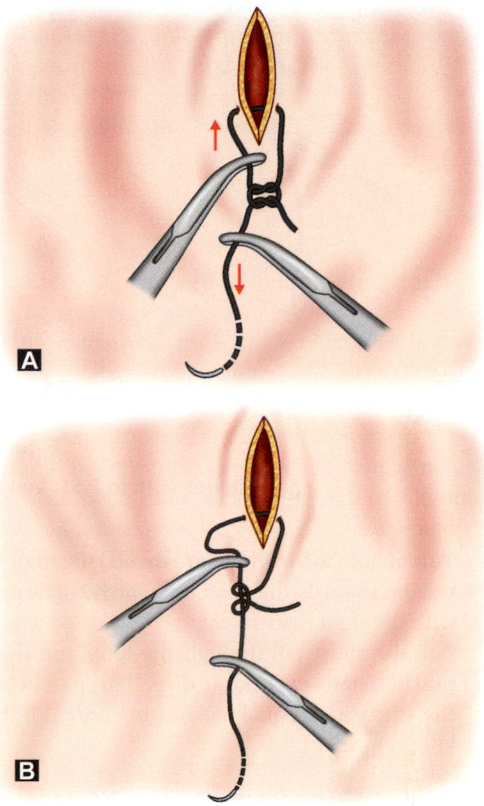

Figures 2.51A and B

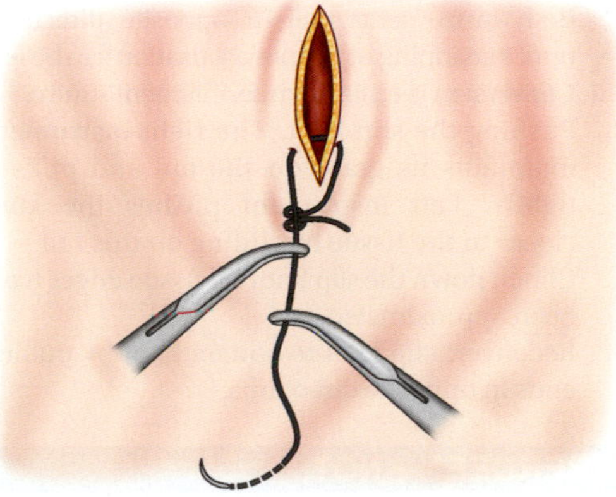

Figure 2.52

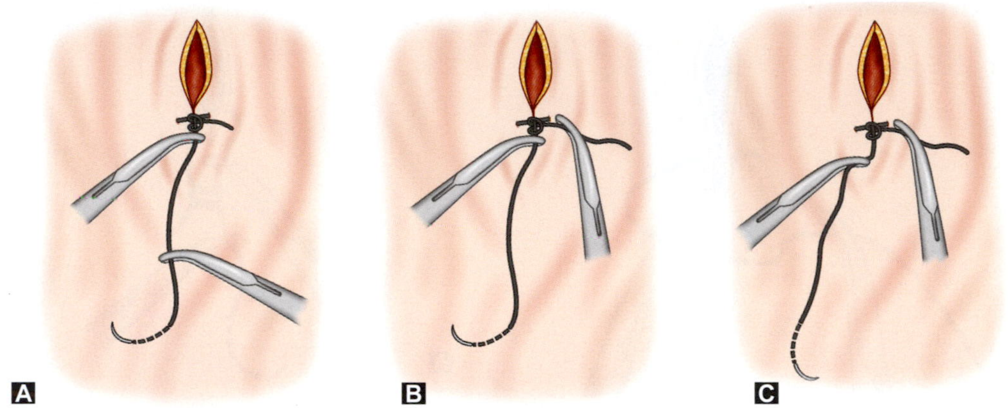

Figures 2.53A to C

Figures 2.46 to 2.53: Various steps of intracorporeal knotting

4. Tips of both instruments are moved together in unison towards the short tail which is grasped with the right instrument.
5. Pull the short tail through the loop and then pull both tails in opposite directions parallel to the stitch with equal tension to configure the knot (Fig. 2.50).

Slip Knot Conversion to the Square Knot (Szabo Technique)

This is essential to tighten the first half knot to provide adequate grip (Figs 2.51 to 2.53).

1. Both instruments grasp the loop on same side one below the knot and one above the knot.
2. Both instruments pull in opposite directions until a snapping or popping sensation can be felt. Conversion is easier in monofilament suture.
3. Pushing the slip knot. The right instrument maintains its grasp on the tail and pulls it tightly. Left instrument pushes the knot closer to the tissue by sliding on this tail.
4. Clinch down the slip knot till tissue edges have been approximated.
5. Reconvert slip knot to square knot by pulling ends in opposite directions.

ABERDEEN KNOT

This knot is applied at the end of a continuous suture, when left with a loop and a free end (Figs 2.54 to 2.58). To tie this knot, loop is displayed

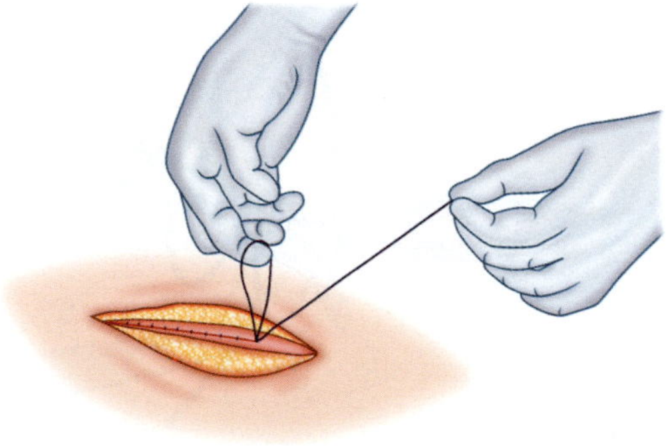

Figure 2.54

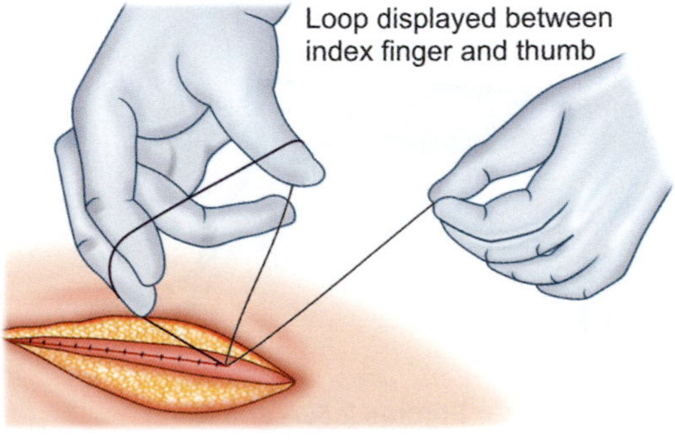

Figure 2.55

between the index finger and thumb of right hand and free end is grasped between the index finger and thumb of the left hand through the loop and by pulling it through and releasing the right hand thread, old loop is eliminated. New loop is formed again between right index finger and thumb and left hand thread is pulled again. Whole process is repeated 6–7 times using 'sea saw' movement. Finally the free end is passed through the loop and tightened down.

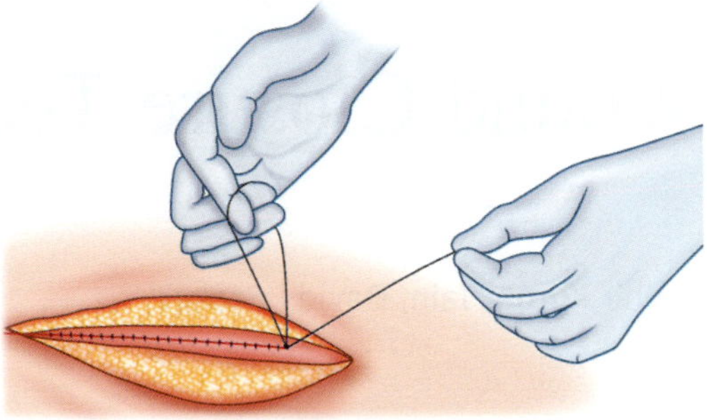

Figure 2.57

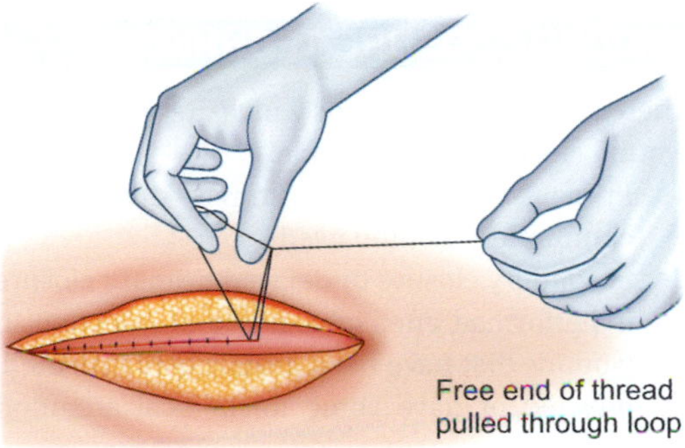

Figure 2.56

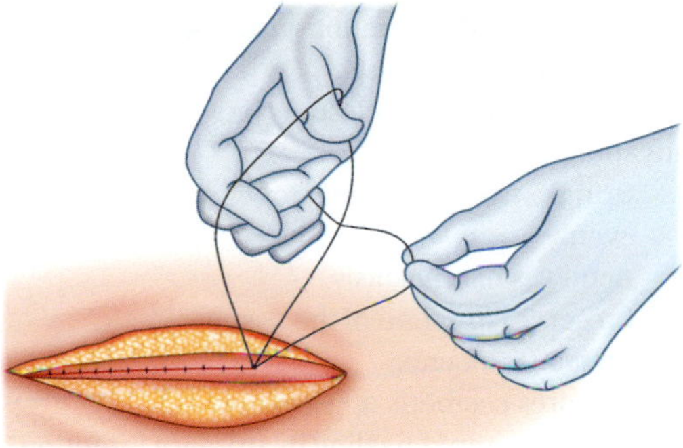

Figure 2.58

Figures 2.54 to 2.58: Various steps of Aberdeen knot tying

Key Points

1. Knots are used for approximation of tissues and ligation of blood vessels.
2. Multifilament sutures are easier to tie than monofilament suture and give a more secure knot.
3. Surgeon's knot or square knot should be used as far as possible.
4. Granny knot should not be used as it is not a safe knot.
5. Whatever type of knot is used the hands should cross after one throw to lock it and make it safe.

Wound Closure Techniques

3

Sudhir Kumar Jain, David L Stoker

The majority of lacerations can be repaired by primary wound closure.

Primary wound closure has the following advantages:

1. Brings wound edges together neatly and evenly
2. Achieves haemostasis
3. Preserves function of the tissue
4. Prevents infection
5. Restores cosmetic appearance
6. Promotes rapid healing by primary intention
7. Decreases patient discomfort and morbidity.

Time of Wound Closure

There is a direct relationship between the time of wound closure and the risk of infection.

Wounds of the face and scalp can be closed by primary closure up to 72 hours after injury without increasing the risk of infection, due to the high vascular supply in this region. In other areas there is no significant time related difference in infection rates for wounds closed within 18 hours.

Increased Risk of Infection

There is a high incidence of wound infection after laceration repair in the following situations:

1. Diabetes mellitus.
2. Obesity.
3. Malnourishment.
4. Immunosuppression, e.g. HIV infection.
5. Patient on steroids, chemotherapeutic agents or immunosuppressive therapy.
6. Crush injuries leading to devitalised tissue.
7. Contaminated wounds.

WOUND CLOSURE TECHNIQUES

There are five main options which are available for wound closure. These include:

1. Primary closure by sutures—this is the commonest method used.
2. Secondary closure or delayed primary closure is performed after taking care of infection in wounds that have been grossly contaminated, infected or have come to medical attention late.
3. Tissue adhesives, e.g. cyanoacrylate glue
4. Staples—skin staples are used in large wounds to save time. They are more expensive, but give an equally good cosmetic result.
5. Surgical tapes or Steri-strips.

In this chapter primary closure by suture will be described.

SUTURING OF LACERATIONS

Suturing of lacerations is generally performed under local anaesthesia except in the following situations which may require general anaesthesia:

1. Large lacerations where the requirement of local anaesthesia will exceed the upper limit of safe dose.
2. Severe contamination requiring extensive cleaning or removal of foreign body or extensive tissue debridement.
3. Open fractures, tendon, nerve or major blood vessel injury.
4. Complex structures requiring meticulous repair, e.g. eyelid.

Equipment Required for Wound Suturing

1. Universal precaution kit.
2. Suturing tray containing needle holder, toothed forceps, and suture scissors.
3. 1 or 2% lignocaine with or without adrenaline for local anaesthesia.
4. 10 cc syringe and 21–25 gauge needles for infiltrating anaesthetic agent.
5. Appropriate sutures.
6. Wound preparation and cleaning materials, e.g. povidone iodine solution, gauze pieces, normal saline.
7. Tetanus immunisation serum.

Steps of Laceration Suturing

1. Wound assessment.
2. Wound preparation.
3. Wound closure.
4. Tetanus prophylaxis.

Wound Assessment

1. Establish approximate time of injury as after four hours, the wound should be scrubbed to remove the protein coagulum.
2. Determine exact mechanism of injury which can point towards an underlying fracture, retained foreign body, tendon or nerve injury or wound contamination.
3. Ask about tetanus immunisation status.
4. Test for distal sensory and motor function to rule out nerve and tendon injury.
5. Consider imaging studies if there is a radio-opaque retained foreign body such as glass.
6. Wound should be accurately described in the patient record as it may have medicolegal consequences or insurance implications.

Wound Preparation

Hair removal may be required for more precise wound closure. However, shaving might introduce infection. Clipping the hair may be a better approach than shaving. Eyebrows are usually not trimmed or shaved because the hair may re-grow in abnormal patterns, and they are a useful guide to correct alignment of a forehead wound.

1. Wound cleaning is done either by direct scrubbing or irrigation of the tissue. Vigorous scrubbing may lead to tissue damage which may increase the risk of infection.
2. Wound irrigation is another method of wound preparation. It can be achieved either by continuous or pulsatile irrigation. Continuous high pressure syringe irrigation significantly reduces the bacterial count, and is particularly useful in densly contaminated tissue with limited vascularity such as a lower extremity wound. Irrigation pressures between 5 and 8 psi are appropriate and can be readily obtained with a 30–60 ml syringe and a 19 gauge needle. High pressure irrigation is contraindicated in a well vascularised location with delicate soft tissues such as eye lid, because it can lead to tissue damage in these areas with an increase in infection rate. A variety of solutions, e.g. detergents, hydrogen peroxide and concentrated Betadine have been used to irrigate wounds, but these are no longer recommended because of their damaging effects on tissues. Normal saline is the solution of choice because it does not damage tissue and is widely available and inexpensive. 100 cc of saline is used for each cm of wound. If using plain Lignocaine for local anaesthesia, buffer by adding 1 ml of sodium bicarbonate to 9 ml of lignocaine to reduce the pain of injection. Inject slowly, and subdermally, beginning inside the cut margin of the wound. Avoid piercing the intact skin. The maximum safe dose of lignocaine is 3 mg/kg. It can be increased to upto 7 mg/kg when Lignocaine is used along with adrenaline.

WOUND SUTURING

Face

Use 4-0 or 5-0 monofilament suture on a cutting needle. Both absorbable and nonabsorbable suture can be used on the face. The type of stitch used is either simple interrupted or subcuticular. Layered closure with a 3-0 or 4-0 polyglactin suture may be needed to approximate the muscle if the wound is deep. Sutures are removed in 5 days.

Scalp

A 2-0 or 3-0 nonabsorbable monofilament suture on a cutting needle is used for suturing. Sutures are removed in 7–10 days.

Lip

A 4-0 or 5-0 synthetic absorbable suture on a tapercut needle is used for the deeper layers and a 3-0 synthetic monofilament on cutting needle is used for the skin. Simple interrupted sutures are applied for deeper layers and for the skin.

Oral Cavity

A 4-0 absorbable gut or synthetic absorbable suture on tapercut needle is used for suturing employing the mattress technique.

TYPES OF SUTURES

Simple Interrupted Suture

This is the most common suture employed for closure of lacerations. A fine smooth non-absorbable suture, e.g. nylon or polypropylene is used for this purpose because it causes much less tissue reaction than silk. Cutting needles are used for applying this suture. The needle should pass at a right angle to the incision line and should pass through the whole thickness of the wound (Fig. 3.1). If the depth of the incised wound is 'X' then needle should pass at a distance of one 'X' from the cut margin of wound and come out at a distance of 'X' from the other margin of the wound, so that the distance between entry and exit point of suture in the skin is '2X' (Fig. 3.2). This rule does not apply to wounds more than 1 cm deep, where layered closure is required.

Sutures should be tied with a tension just enough to approximate the edges without causing tissue constriction. If sutures are tied too tightly they will cause ischemia, delayed healing and increased scarring. Knots should be placed laterally and away from the wound. The next stitch should be placed at a distance of '2X' from the previous stitch (Fig. 3.2). When cutting sutures, the length of left out tails from knot should be just less than 1 cm. If the tails are too long they will entangle with the next stitch, and if tails are left too short, there is a danger of knot slippage and difficulty in suture removal later on. Sutures are generally removed around the 7th day except in the face where they are removed on the 5th day. Below the knee and on the back, sutures are left for 10–14 days to prevent wound dehiscence.

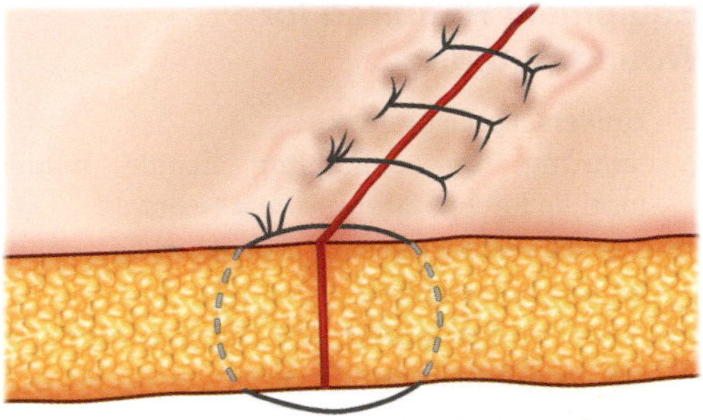

Figure 3.1: Suture should be placed at right angle to the wound edge and should traverse whole thickness of the wound

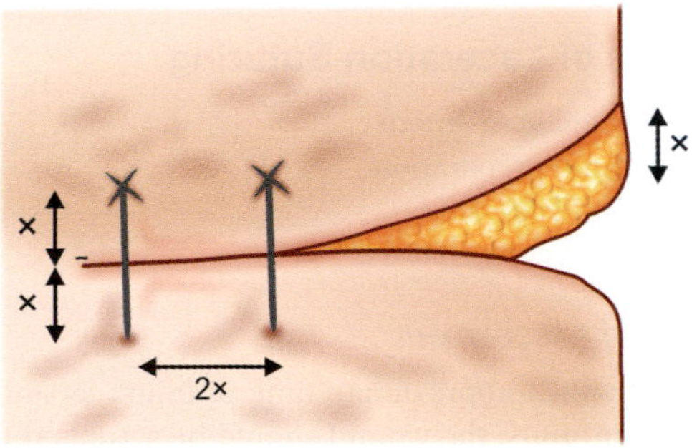

Figure 3.2: Bite should be at a distance of X from the wound margin and come out at a distance of X from the opposite wound margin. X is the thickness of the wound. Distance between two sutures should be '2X'

Vertical Mattress Suture (Fig. 3.3)

This suture is commonly used for closing surgical wounds. It is useful if there is excess skin or loose subcutaneous fat. There are two entry and two exit points. All points lie in the same line. Firstly, the needle enters the skin at a right angle at a distance

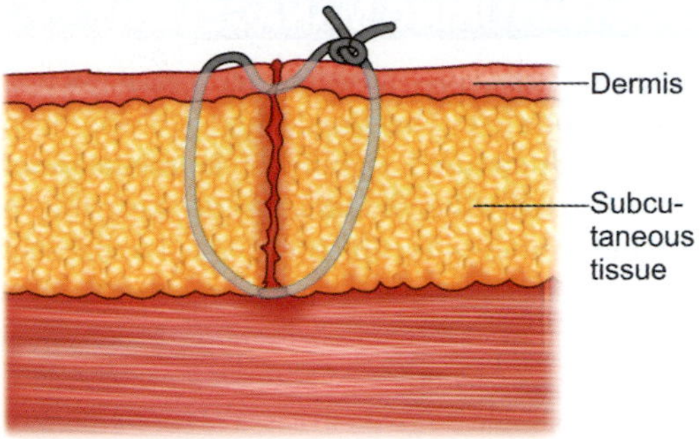

Figure 3.3: Method of taking vertical mattress suture

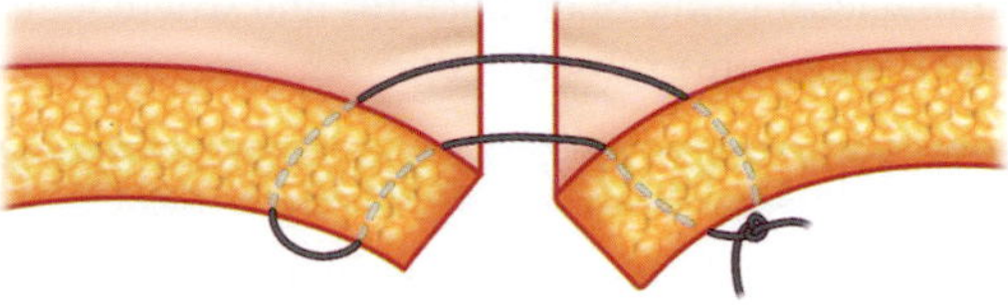

Figure 3.4: Inversion of skin edges by vertical mattress suture

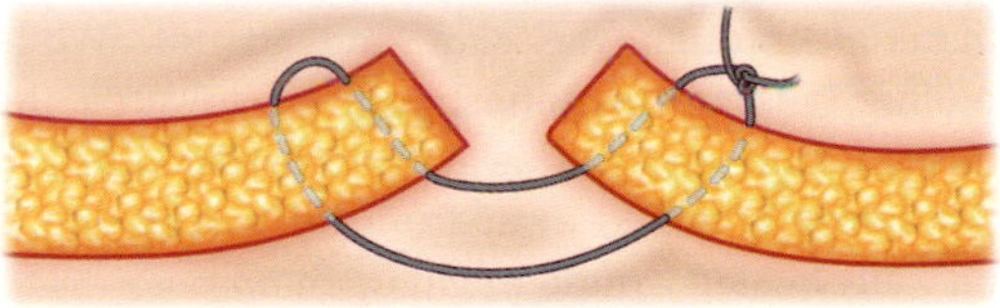

Figure 3.5: Eversion of skin margin by vertical mattress suture

from the wound margin of 'X' (depth of wound) or about 1 cm if a wound is deep and a layered closure has been performed. It traverses the whole thickness of the wound, and the needle comes out from the other side of the wound at a distance of 'X' or 1 cm. Secondly, the direction of needle is reversed. The needle is placed close to the margin of the wound, traversing epidermis only in such a manner that all four points lie in same line, and the skin edges are everted. The knot is tied to one side (Figs 3.4 and 3.5).

Horizontal Mattress Suture (Figs 3.6 and 3.7)

This is another eversion suture, and may be used where the skin is thick, for example on the sole of the foot. There are again two entry and two exit

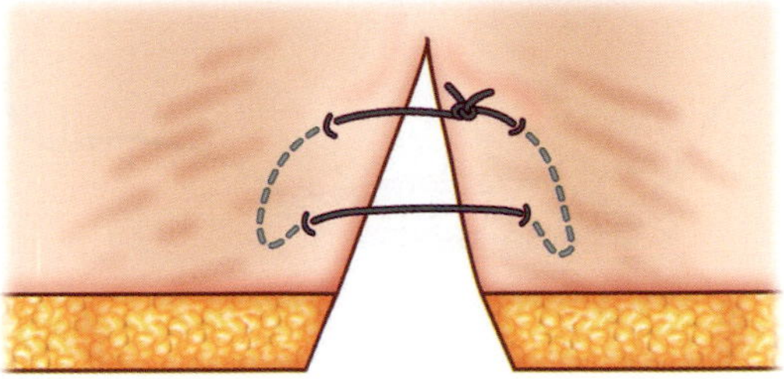

Figure 3.6: Horizontal mattress suture

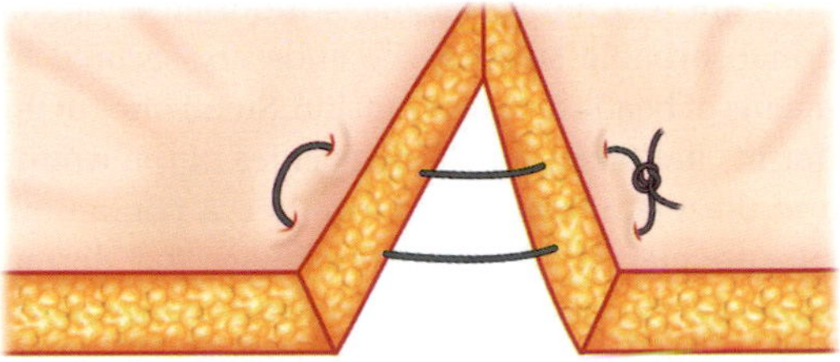

Figure 3.7: Eversion of skin margin by horizontal mattress suture

points. Firstly, the needle is placed 4 to 8 mm from the wound edge. It then passes through to the opposite wound edge, where it exits the skin at about the same distance on the other side of the wound edge. The needle is reversed using the needle holder and forceps, inserted into the same skin edge 4 to 8 mm further down the wound, and passed from this side back to the other side of the wound. The needle exits the skin about 4 to 8 mm down the original wound edge from the initial insertion site. This suture is shown in Figures 3.6 and 3.7. The main problem with this suture is that skin which is caught between each horizontal bite may lose its circulation when the knot is tied. These areas of ischaemia may extend up to 50% of the entire skin margin as further sutures are placed. Partial necrosis of the skin margin is therefore quite common.

Subcuticular Suture (Fig. 3.8)

This suture gives a very fine and neat scar because approximation of skin margins is perfect. Either

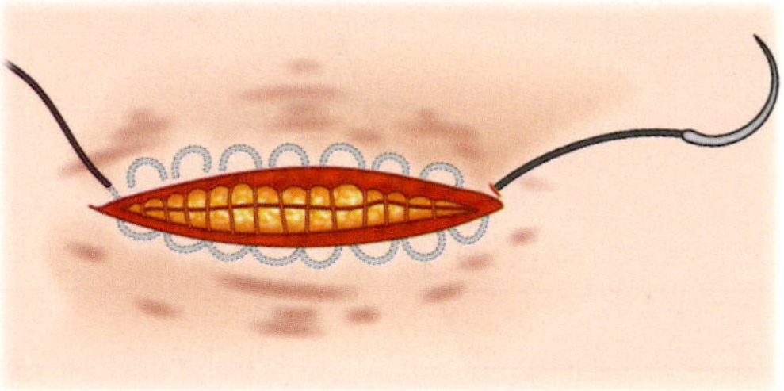

Figure 3.8: Subcuticular suture

absorbable or nonabsorbable suture can be used for this technique. For absorbable sutures, the ends are secured by means of a buried knot. For nonabsorbable sutures, the ends are secured by means of beads or a knot outside. Small bites of the dermis are taken on alternate sides of the wound and these are then pulled together. A continuous subcuticular suture to approximate the dermal layer of the skin is a fast and cosmetically satisfactory method of skin closure. Its main advantage is that additional scarring from sutures is avoided. Its drawback is that it gives no support to the underlying tissue. Surgical gut should not be used for this suture as it produces an intense tissue reaction. If other synthetic absorbable sutures are used, knots should be placed deep and well away from the wound edge. A nonabsorbable nylon or prolene is ideal. Long wounds should have intermittent bridges or external loops of suture to facilitate suture removal. This suture should not be used where there is increased potential for wound infection, as it is not possible to open a part of the wound by removing one or two interrupted sutures.

POSTSUTURING MANAGEMENT

Cover wounds after suturing for 1–2 days with loose protective covering. This protects from contamination until significant epithelialisation has occurred. After 2 days, gentle cleansing of sutured wound is acceptable. Topical application of antibiotic ointment or petroleum jelly may allow increased rate of epithelialisation. Prophylactic antibiotics are not indicated after a simple laceration repair but should be given in cases of contamination (including animal or human bites), crush wounds, and in diabetic patients. Antibiotics are also indicated in oral lacerations, open fractures and where joints and tendons are exposed.

SUTURE REMOVAL

Sutures should be cut as close as possible to the point where it emerges from the skin on the side of incision opposite to the knot (Fig. 3.9A). This enables the surgeon to draw the minimal length of the exposed and possibly contaminated suture material through the skin and tissues. While pulling, suture traction should be towards the incision line, and not away from it (Fig. 3.9B). If the suture is pulled away from the suture line, a partially healed wound might open up.

OTHER METHODS OF WOUND CLOSURE

Tissue Adhesives

These adhesives consist of a liquid monomer made by a combination of formaldehyde and

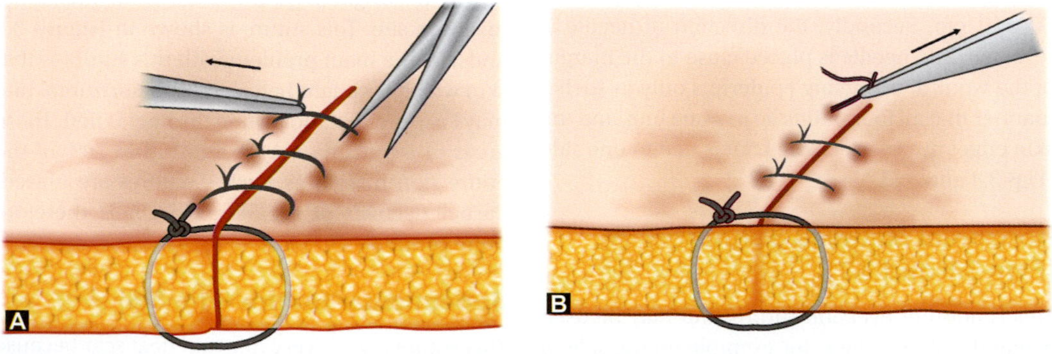

Figures 3.9A and B: Proper method of suture removal

cyanoacrylate. This reacts with hydroxyl ions found in water and blood, thereby causing a reaction which bonds the edges of the skin. The benefits of tissue adhesive include less pain and quick application. They are therefore potentially useful in children. Infection rates are higher with tissue adhesives. For application of a tissue adhesive, skin edges should be approximated closely and a thin layer of adhesive evenly applied. If there is a significant tension during manual approximation, a tissue adhesive should not be used. They should not be applied over areas of high tension such as over joints or in the hand. If wrongly applied they can be easily removed with acetone, petroleum jelly or antibacterial ointment. They have some antibacterial property against gram-positive bacteria.

Staples

The benefit of skin staples includes fast application, lower rate of foreign body reaction and decreased infection rate. Staples are particularly useful for wound closure in the scalp, extremities and trunk wounds. They are also commonly used on long surgical incisions. Their use saves time.

Surgical or Adhesive Tapes (Steri-Strips)

These cause little skin reactivity, and are useful for very small wounds, and in children. If additional adhesive solution is required, Opsite spray is ideal, as tincture of Benzoic acid may lead to a local skin reaction or even wound infection. Tapes are not ideal for primary closure of wounds, but can be placed after suture removal and may decrease skin tension. They usually fall away in 7–10 days.

Key Points

1. Majority of wounds should be closed primarily to achieve optimum cosmetic results and for preservation of function.
2. Wounds should be closed within 18 hours to avoid wound infection except for wounds of face and scalp where a delay of up to 72 hours is acceptable.
3. Wound preparation by hair removal and irrigation by normal saline with irrigation pressure of 5–8 psi is mandatory before wound closure.
4. Povidone iodine and hydrogen peroxide should be avoided for wound irrigation as they have a damaging effect on tissue.
5. As far as possible simple interrupted suture should be applied.
6. A vertical mattress should be used if there is excess of skin or loose subcutaneous fat.
7. A horizontal mattress may be useful for either eversion or inversion of a wound edge but there is a higher incidence of ischaemia and necrosis of the skin.
8. A subcuticular suture gives a very fine and neat scar but has the disadvantage of not providing any support to the deep tissues

Surgery of Common Skin Lesions Under Local Anaesthesia

4

Sudhir Kumar Jain, Beryl Antoinette De Souza

The indications for removal of skin lesions are as follows:

1. Suspicion of malignancy.
2. Cosmetic reasons.
3. If the lesion is hampering the function of a joint or causing compression of a neurovascular structure.
4. To avoid complications such as infection, bleeding, pain or irritation.

If a particular lesion is being removed for cosmetic reasons, all efforts should be made to give a neat scar, which is less conspicuous than the original contour of the lesion. Other options for treatment like use of lasers, cryosurgery, electrocautery excision, curettage or local application of skin ointments should be discussed with the patient before offering excision. An accurate clinical diagnosis and dermatology input may be required in these cases. Lasers are particularly useful in arteriovenous malformations and the skin lesions of neurofibromatosis, i.e. café-au-lait spots.

ANAESTHESIA

The majority of skin lesions can be removed under local anaesthesia. This can be in the form of local infiltration or a nerve block, e.g. digital, brachial, intercostal or femoral nerve block or a field block (Figs 4.1 to 4.3). The following agents are commonly used for local anaesthesia:

Lignocaine 0.5% prepared from 1 or 2% commercially available solutions by dilution with normal saline is generally used. Maximum dose is 3 mg/kg of body weight without adrenaline and

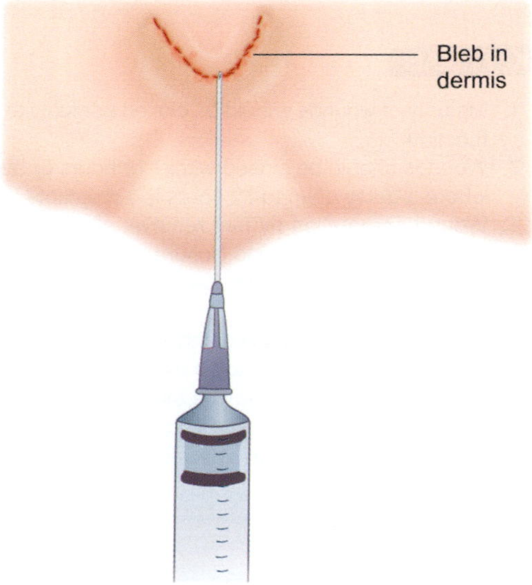

Figure 4.1: A bleb should be raised in the dermis by a 24 number needle before starting infiltration of local anaesthesia

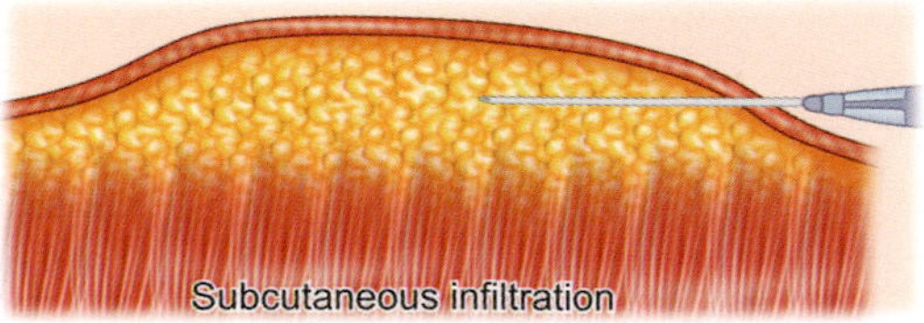

Figure 4.2: Method of infiltration of local anaesthesia in subcutaneous plane

7 mg/kg body weight with adrenaline. Lignocaine 1 or 2% with 1:200,000 adrenaline gives a longer period of anaesthesia because anaesthetic washout from the tissues is delayed due to arteriolar constriction. A delay in absorption permits use of lower doses of the anaesthetic. Local vasoconstriction also reduces the capillary oozing in the operative field. An adrenaline containing solution should not be used in the vicinity of end arteries because vasoconstriction can endanger blood supply particularly in the fingers, toes, ear lobule, tip of the nose and the penis.

Bupivacaine 0.5% or 0.25% solution is available with or without adrenaline. It is a longer acting agent, but slower in onset of action. Its effect can last up to 6–8 hours, giving a significantly better postoperative pain relief. Injection of local anaesthetic agent into skin can be more painful than the surgery itself. 50:50 mixtures of lignocaine and bupivacaine may be used for both quick initial effect, and long acting pain relief.

Ways to minimise pain during injection of local anaesthetic include:

- Explanation of the procedure to the patient with reassurance to allay anxiety is very important.
- Topical application of local anaesthetic cream (a combination of lignocaine and prilocaine) avoids pain during infiltration of tissues.
- Pre-warming the solution along with the addition of bicarbonate (0.5 ml in 9.5 ml of lignocaine) makes it less acidic.
- Slow injection into subcutaneous tissue first.
- Initial epidermal infiltration by raising a wheal with a fine (26 G) needle, prior to using a large (19 G) needle for main infiltration decreases discomfort to a great extent.

Field Block (Fig. 4.3)

In this method the local anaesthetic agent is injected into the tissues at some distance from the actual site of operation, so that a zone of anaesthesia is created surrounding the operation area. The skin can be anaesthetised first in the area of the block using a small fine needle. The block itself may require a long needle. Injection is made into the subcutaneous plane, and before infiltrating the deeper planes, the syringe should

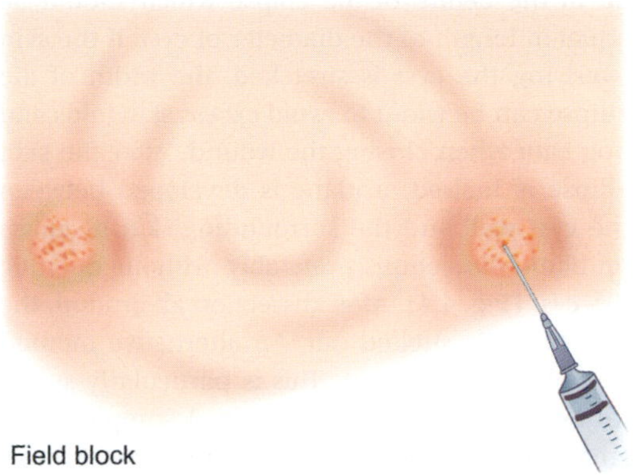

Figure 4.3: Field block method of local anaesthesia

be aspirated to make sure that the needle has not entered a blood vessel. During injection the needle is gradually withdrawn. The advantage of a field block is that the lesion is not obscured by local swelling.

Nerve Block

Local anaesthetic agent can be injected around a nerve to anaesthetise the area which it serves. Digital nerve block is commonly employed for surgery on fingers or toes. Plain lignocaine is injected at the base of the digit on both sides to block the dorsal and palmar digital nerves. Injection is made in the web space on both sides of the finger. The needle is pushed vertically down until it touches bone, then it is slightly withdrawn and local anaesthetic is injected after confirmation by aspiration that the needle is not in a vessel. 0.5–1 ml of 0.5% lignocaine is often sufficient on each side.

COMMON SKIN PROCEDURES

Excision of Sebaceous Cyst

Excision of sebaceous cyst is advised due to its tendency to grow and become infected. The cyst should be excised completely in order to avoid recurrence. If the cyst is small and the overlying skin is healthy, a linear incision is employed. If the cyst is markedly protuberant or if the skin is thin and unhealthy or if there is an overlying punctum, an elliptical incision is used. The punctum should be in the centre of the ellipse which should be equal in length to the diameter of cyst. If the skin overlying the cyst is stretched, the width of the ellipse can be wider to avoid excess skin folds and dog ears when closing the wound. After the skin ellipse is incised, a plane is developed between the cyst wall and the surrounding skin by sharp or blunt dissection, preferably without opening the cyst (Fig. 4.4). After dissection all around, the cyst is easily shelled out. An alternative method is avulsion of the cyst. This is particularly suited for removal of cysts on the scalp. A comparatively small incision is required and cutaneous scarring is less. A skin flap is raised on only one side. The cyst is then deliberately opened and contents squeezed out. Using a pair of nontoothed dissecting forceps with one blade outside the cyst and one blade inside, the cyst wall is grasped at its deepest part (Fig. 4.5) and by traction on the forceps, the entire cyst wall can be avulsed easily. The cyst wall is held at the deepest portion because the deeper part is tougher than the superficial portion and will not tear easily. The wound is sutured and a pressure dressing is applied to prevent haematoma formation in the cavity.

If the sebaceous cyst is infected, removal is deferred until the inflammation subsides. If there is abscess formation, it should be incised and pus drained. Curettage of the abscess cavity or swabbing with pure carbolic acid may prevent the cyst from reforming. Infected sebaceous cysts should not be excised as wound complication rates are high and the resulting scars are unsatisfactory.

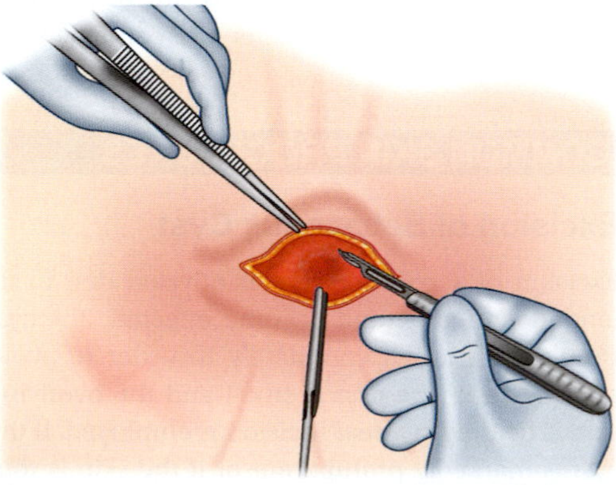

Figure 4.4: Raising flaps for excision of sebaceous cyst

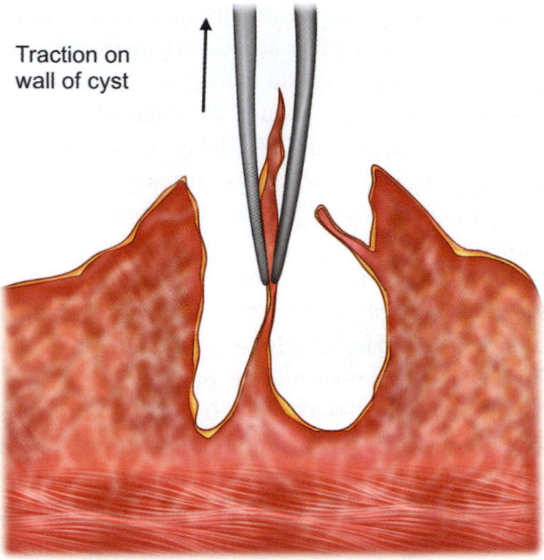

Figure 4.5: Avulsion method of removal of sebaceous cyst

They often do not recur after incision because infection frequently destroys the lining of the cyst.

LIPOMA EXCISION

Lipomas are slowly growing benign connective tissue tumours derived from adult type fat cells. They can occur anywhere in the body and are therefore known as universal tumours. However they seldom occur in eyelids, pinna or penis. They should be excised if they are rapidly enlarging, painful, unsightly or if there is a concern about malignant change or there are associated secondary changes, e.g. myxomatous degeneration, traumatic fat necrosis (suggested by lipoma hardening after trauma) or calcification. Malignant change is suggested by rapid growth over 6–8 weeks, firmness, or early fixity to surrounding tissue. Retroperitoneal lipoma, large lipoma in the thigh or lipomas of shoulder region are more likely to undergo malignant change. They may rarely hamper movement.

For a subcutaneous lipoma excision, a skin incision is deepened through the overlying fat until the capsule of the lipoma is reached. It can be differentiated from the surrounding fat by larger fat globules, colour, and a fine capsule. The lesion can often be enucleated after incision of its fine capsule, but larger lesions may need sharp dissection. If a lipoma is adherent to the underlying muscle it should not be removed under local anaesthetic as there may be deep extensions between muscle bellies, with involvement of neurovascular bundles. If a deeper lesion is suspected or if the lesion is more than 5 cm in diameter, a CT or MRI scan is indicated for accurate anatomical delineation.

BASAL CELL CARCINOMA (RODENT ULCER)

Basal cell carcinoma should be excised with 2 mm of normal tissue all around, on all aspects including the deeper plane. Completeness of excision should be verified by histopathology.

Complete excision is associated with a recurrence rate of less than 2%. Moh has described a technique for recurrent lesions to ensure complete tumour excision. This technique essentially comprises of excision in layers with horizontal frozen section control. Radiotherapy is an alternative to surgical excision in difficult situations like infiltrating lesion of eyes, nose or mouth which would otherwise require major reconstruction after complete excision.

SQUAMOUS CELL CARCINOMA

These should be completely excised with 1 cm of macroscopically normal skin. Skin flaps should be extensively raised so that a still larger area of deep fascia can be excised. This tumour is sensitive to radiotherapy which may be used as an alternative or as an adjunct to surgery.

MALIGNANT MELANOMA

If a malignant melanoma is suspected, the initial surgery should be carried out to excise the lesion with margins reflecting the tumour depth. For a tumour excised with < 1 mm depth, a wide excision of 1 cm margin around the tumour is sufficient. If the tumour is between 1–2 mm in depth, a 1–2 cm wide margin is adequate. For tumours > 2 mm in depth, a 2 cm clearance is recommended. The excision should be carried down to but not through the deep fascia. All patients with tumour depth of > 1 cm should be offered sentinel node biopsy at the same time as the wide excision. If the sentinel node is positive then the patient will need to undergo complete nodal clearance.

Key Points

1. Common indications for removal of skin lesion are cosmetic, concern about malignancy, bothersome symptoms or limitation in the movement or function of a joint.
2. Majority of skin lesions can be removed under local anaesthesia.
3. Sebaceous cyst should be removed if there is tendency to grow or if it becomes infected.
4. Sebaceous cyst should be removed completely to avoid recurrence.
5. Basal cell carcinoma is excised with 2 mm of normal tissue all around.
6. Squamous cell carcinoma is excised with 1 cm of normal skin.
7. Malignant melanoma should be excised by an experienced surgeon.

Sutures in Surgery

5

Sudhir Kumar Jain, David L Stoker

DEFINITION

The word "suture" describes any material which is used to ligate blood vessels, tubular structures and ducts or to approximate tissues and close wounds. The use of sutures dates back to the era of the great Indian surgeon Sushruta, the father of ancient Indian surgery. In 2000 BC, Egyptians and Syrians used sutures for various purposes. All sorts of materials ranging from horse hair, animal tendons, wire, silk, cotton and linen, have been used as suture materials. Some of these are still used today. In the modern era, technical advances have brought us to a stage where specific sutures are available for a particular use.

IDEAL SUTURE

Till date no available suture material meets all requirements but an ideal suture should have the following properties:

1. It should be devoid of any allergic, carcinogenic, capillary or electrostatic action.
2. It should be easy to sterilise.
3. It should not produce any magnetic field around it, as it happens in a steel wire.
4. It should be easy to handle.
5. It should cause minimal tissue reaction.
6. It should not promote growth of bacteria around it, in other words it should be resistant to infection.
7. It should have favourable tensile strength and hold the tissue securely throughout the phase of wound healing.
8. It should absorb with minimal tissue reaction after having served its purpose.
9. It should have high tensile strength.
10. It should hold tissue securely when knotted without cutting or fraying the tissue.

CLASSIFICATION OF SUTURE MATERIAL (TABLE 5.1)

Suture Size

Suture size denotes the diameter of the suture material. Suture size is generally denoted by 0's. As the number of "0's" in the suture size increase, diameter of suture strand decreases. Suture size is directly proportional to the tensile strength of the suture. The smaller the size of the suture, the less is the tensile strength of the suture.

Knot Tensile Strength

This is measured by the force, in pounds, which the suture can withstand before it breaks when knotted. Tensile strength of the tissue is measured by its ability to withstand stress. Tensile strength of the suture should always exceed the tensile strength of the tissue.

Sutures can be classified in many ways:

1. Monofilament versus multifilament
2. Absorbable versus nonabsorbable
3. Natural versus synthetic.

Table 5.1: Classification of sutures
1. Absorbable
• ***Natural***
– Surgical gut (plain or chromic)
– Collagen (plain or chromic)
• ***Synthetic***
– Poliglecaprone 25
– Polydioxanone
– Polyglycolic acid
– Polyglactin 910
– Polycaprolactone
– Polysorb
– Maxon
– V-Loc™
– Caprosyn
2. Nonabsorbable
• ***Natural***
– Surgical silk
– Surgical linen
– Cotton
– Surgical steel
• ***Synthetic***
– Polyamide
– Polypropylene
– Polyester
– Nylon
– Polybutester suture
– Coated polybutester
– Surgipro II™

Monofilament versus Multifilament

Monofilament sutures comprising a single strand of material, encounter less resistance when passing through tissue, and provide poor habitat for harbouring organisms. This property makes them suitable for use in vascular surgery. They are easy to tie, but are delicate and can get broken easily. They are also more amenable to crushing or crimping.

Multifilament sutures consist of multiple filaments and strands, twisted and braided together. They may be coated for smooth passage through tissue. They have more tensile strength, pliability and flexibility. They are well suited for intestinal anastomosis.

Absorbable versus Nonabsorbable Sutures

Sutures which undergo rapid degradation in tissue, losing their tensile strength within 60 days are known as absorbable sutures. Those which maintain their tensile strength for more than 60 days are known as nonabsorbable sutures. Silk loses 50% of its tensile strength in one year and has no strength at the end of two years. Nylon loses 25% of its original strength during two years. Cotton retains 30–40% of its original strength at the end of two years.

ABSORBABLE SUTURES

These are either derived from collagen or synthetic polymers.

Catgut Sutures

These are either derived from the submucosa of sheep intestine or from serosa of beef intestine. Collagenous tissue obtained from gut is treated with an aldehyde solution for cross-linking, which gives the suture more strength and makes it resistant to enzymatic degradation. Sutures obtained in this way are known as plain gut. If plain gut is additionally treated by chromium trioxide, it is known as chromic gut. Chromic gut has more cross linkage and is more resistance to absorption. Reabsorption of gut is by enzymatic degradation, mainly by the lysosomal enzyme acid phosphatase initially, followed by leucine aminopeptidase. Collagenase also plays a significant role in degradation. Plain gut is rapidly absorbed and maintains its tensile strength for 7–10 days and is completely absorbed in 70 days. Tensile strength of chromic gut is maintained for 14–20 days. Drawbacks of gut suture are breakage during knot tying and variation in retention of tensile strength. There is also a growing concern regarding transfer of Prion disease.

Collagen Sutures

These are derived from homogenised tendo-Achilles of beef cattle and are 100% pure collagen. They are available in plain and chromic form. They are stiffer than surgical gut. Therefore handling becomes difficult in a large size suture. Finer size sutures are used in eye surgery.

Fascia Lata

This is obtained from the thigh muscles of beef cattle. It used to be used for hernia repair. It is still occasionally used for surgical correction of drooping upper eye lid and for facial palsy.

Kangaroo Tendon

This is obtained from tail tendons of small Kangaroos and varies in length from 10 inches to 18 inches. It has a high tensile strength.

Synthetic Polymer Sutures

Synthetic polymer sutures available are:

1. Polyglycolic acid suture (Homomer)
2. Copolymers of glycolide and lactide (Polyglactin)
3. Poliglecaprone 25 (Monocryl)
4. Polydioxanone prepared from polyester.

Polyglycolic Acid Suture (Dexon™, Dexon 1™)

This is a homomer of polyglycolic acid. It has high tensile strength with retention of 60% strength at day 7, and 35% at day 60. This suture is completely hydrolysed by 90–120 days. This is a multifilament suture with good handling quality and knot security. It has a high coefficient of friction, which gives rise to drag during passage through tissue. This suture has high tissue reactivity and may potentiate infection. To minimise tissue drag, a coated form of polyglycolic acid is available. Coating is in the form of copolymer of glycolide and epsilon caprolactone (Dexon 1™).

*Polyglactin (Vicryl™)**

This is a copolymer of glycolic acid and lactic acid. Polyglactin 910 consists of glycolide and lactide in the ratio of 9:1. For every nine parts of glycolic acid there is one part of lactic acid. The lactide element is more hydrophobic than glycolic acid, and thus slows down the absorption of water by suture material, and hence the breakdown of linkage of copolymer chain is slowed down. Vicryl comes with a coating of 50% polyglactin and 50% calcium stearate. This polyglactin coating consist of 35% glycolide and 65% lactide and is known as polyglactin 370. Calcium stearate is an absorbable organic lubricant. Coating of polyglactin 370 and calcium stearate over polyglactin 910 reduces the surface friction of the suture thus avoiding tissue drag and premature locking. There is minimal absorption till 40 days. After 40 days there is rapid absorption and the suture completely disappears between 56–70 days. If coated polyglactin 910 is exposed to gamma irradiation, it results in a low molecular weight suture in comparison to coated polyglactin and is available as vicryl rapidae. Vicryl rapidae has 30% less tensile strength than coated vicryl. Coated vicryl retains 80% of postimplantation tensile strength at 14 days, and 30% of tensile strength at 21 days. Vicryl rapidae loses all its tensile strength between 10 and 12 days. Vicryl rapidae is totally absorbed within 42 days.

For Secure Knotting of Vicryl

There should be a double throw in the first half knot, followed by additional two throws (Total of four throws). Ends should be cut long. Coated Vicryl sutures are suitable for use any where except in the neural or cardiovascular tissue. Coated vicryl rapidae suture is well suited for skin closure, episiotomy closure and closure of lacerations under plaster casts. Coated vicryl plus is an antibacterial suture that is covered with a layer of antibacterial agent Triclosan. The antibacterial agent coating offers protection against bacterial colonisation of the suture.

Polydioxanone Suture (PDS and PDS II™)

This monofilament synthetic suture comprises of polyester poly (p-dioxanone). It is a soft, pliable suture and provides support to tissue for 6 weeks. It elicits only slight tissue reaction. It is absorbed through hydrolysis. It retains 70% of tensile strength at 2 weeks, and 50% tensile strength at 4 weeks and 25% at 6 weeks. Absorption is minimal until about the 90th day and is essentially complete within 6 months. It has more flexibility than polyglycolic acid or polyglactin suture.

Poliglecaprone 25 (Monocryl™)

This is a monofilament suture, which has superior pliability for easy handling and tying. It is a copolymer of glycolide and epsilon-caprolactone. It is composed of 75% glycolide and 25% caprolactone and is available in undyed and dyed violet form. This is the most pliable synthetic absorbable suture. It has a smooth surface which passes through tissue with ease. It is virtually inert, and has good tensile strength. It retains 50–60% of its strength at 7th day. All its tensile strength is lost in 21 days. It is absorbed by the mechanism of hydrolysis in 90–120 days.

Polysorb™

It is a braided absorbable suture produced from Lactomer copolymer. Lactomer copolymer consists of glycolide and lactide in ratio of 9:1. Glycolide provides initial high tensile strength in tissue but undergoes hydrolysis rapidly. Lactide has a slower and controlled rate of hydrolysis and gives prolonged tensile strength in tissue. Knot construction is easy with polysorb because knot breaking strength of polysorb is significantly greater than polyglactin 910. Surface of polysorb suture is coated with mixture of caprolactone/glycolide polymer to reduce coefficient of friction.

V-Loc™

It is a barbed suture developed by Covidien Inc. It is self-anchoring and does not need knotting for wound closure. This suture consists of axially barbed segments of size 0 polydioxanone. At the midpoint of each side of axially barbed fibre there is change in direction. The V-Loc™ wound closure device eliminates the need to tie knots, so one can close incisions up to 50% faster without compromising strength and security. It has potential to reduce knot-related complications. The devices use a unidirectional barbed thread which fixates itself in the tissue, with a loop at the start of the thread which anchors it securely at the edge of the wound. Standard suturing techniques can be used, but without the need to tie knots to fixate the suture. The V-Loc™ device provides evenly-spaced barbs throughout the strand, providing secure closure of the incision by distributing tension across the wound.

Caprosyn

It is rapidly absorbing monofilament absorbable suture prepared from polyglactone 621 synthetic polyester. It is made up of glycolide, caprolactone, trimethylene carbonate and lactide. It retains 50–60% knot strength at 5 days after surgery and minimum of 20–30% at 10th postoperative day. There is total loss of tensile strength by 21 days. It has superior handling qualities in comparison to chromic catgut. It is much easier to reposition the knotted caprosyn.

NONABSORBABLE SUTURES

Nonabsorbable sutures are classified into three classes:

Class I	Silk or synthetic fibres of monofilament (twisted or braided)
Class II	Cotton or linen fibres
Class III	Metal wire of monofilament or multifilament construction.

Silk

Silk sutures are nonabsorbable, sterile, and nonmutagenic, consisting of natural proteinacious silk fibers called fibroin. This protein is derived from the domestic silk worm *Bombyx mori*. Silk fibers are treated to remove the naturally occurring sericin gum.

Silk sutures are braided around a core and coated with wax to reduce capillary action. They are colored black with logwood extract. Silk, being a foreign protein, causes more tissue reaction than synthetic nonabsorbable sutures. Silk induces a polymorphonuclear type of cellular reaction. Although classified as nonabsorbable it behaves as a very slowly absorbing suture. It loses most of its tensile strength in about one year and usually cannot be detected in tissues after two years. Encapsulation of the silk with a fibrous capsule occurs in 14–21 days. Handling properties are good, and it knots easily and securely. Surgical silk loses tensile strength when exposed to moisture and should be used dry.

Linen

This is made from flax and is a cellulose material. It is twisted to form a fiber to make a suture. Tissue reaction is similar to silk, and handling and knotting properties are very good. It is unique in the property that it gains 10% more tensile strength when wet. It is still widely used for tying pedicles and as a ligature.

Cotton

It is derived from the hairs of the seeds of the cotton plant. It comprises of twisted, long, staple cotton fibers to form a suture. It retains 50% tensile strength at 6 months and 30–40% tensile strength at 2 years. It gets encapsulated within the body tissue. It is weak in comparison to linen and is rarely used.

Surgical Steel Suture

It is made up of stainless steel (Iron-Chromium-Nickel-Molybdenum alloy). It is available in monofilament and twisted multifilament form. It has high tensile strength with little loss over passage of time. It holds knots well and does not show any tissue reaction. Surgical steel can be used in sternum closure, abdominal wall closure and orthopaedic surgery. Surgical steel is difficult to handle because of its tendency to get kinked, fragmented and barbed. It can pull, cut or tear tissues of the patient.

Nylon

This is composed of a long chain of polyamide polymers. It has a high tensile strength and low tissue reactivity. Because of its elasticity it is well suited for abdominal and skin closure. Nylon has a low coefficient of friction and tissue reaction is minimal. It loses 25% of tensile strength in 1 year. It has a memory and knot security is lower than that of other sutures. It is available as monofilament (Ethilon™) or multifilament strands known as Nurolen. Monofilament nylon in a wet state is more pliable than dry nylon. Multifilament nylon sutures have more strength and elicit less tissue reaction than silk. Multifilament nylon sutures generally lose 15 to 20% of their tensile strength per year in tissue by hydroxylation.

Polyester Fibre

This comprises of untreated fibres of polyester braided into a multifilament strand. This is also known as terylene or dacron. It has a very high tensile strength and relatively low tissue reactivity. It retains tensile strength for an indefinite period. It has become the suture of choice for cardiovascular procedures, blood vessel anastomosis and for placement of prosthetic material. Polyester sutures have a tendency to cut through tissue and to obviate this tendency, coating of Teflon or polybutylate is provided over the polyester suture. Polyester coated with polybutylate is known as Ethibond. The polybutylate coating does not increase the diameter of the suture in contrast to teflon coating and also does not flake in the tissue.

Polypropylene

This is also known as prolene. It is monofilament and has extremely high tensile strength which is retained for indefinite period. It has very low tissue reactivity. It can stretch up to 30% before breaking and hence is useful in situations where postoperative swelling is anticipated. Knotting is extremly secure because the suture deforms on knotting and allows the knot to bend down on itself. It has a low coefficient of friction and slides through tissue readily. In comparison to silk it is less thrombogenic. It is very smooth and does not saw through the tissues. As it does not adhere to tissue, it is useful as a "pull out" suture, e.g. subcuticular suture. Polypropylene is recommended for use where minimal suture reaction is desired, such as in contaminated and infected wounds to minimize sinus formation and suture extrusion.

Polybutester

The Polybutester suture (Novafil™) is a copolymer that comprises of butylene terephthalate (84%) and polytetramethylene ether glycol terephthalate (16%). Polybutester suture has unique performance characteristics. This is a monofilament synthetic nonabsorbable suture. This suture yields significantly greater elongation than other sutures even with low forces and has elasticity which is superior to that of other sutures, allowing the suture to return to its original length once the load is removed.

The Polybutester skin suture diminishes the risk of hypertrophic scar formation because of its special properties allowing it to adapt to changing tensions in the wound. The clinical performance of Polybutester suture has been enhanced by coating its surface with a unique absorbable polymer of polytribolate (Vascufil™).

This polymer is composed of three compounds: glycolide, e-caprolactone, and poloxamer 188. Coating the polybutester suture markedly reduces its drag forces in musculoaponeurotic, colonic, and vascular tissue. Knot security with the Vascufil™ suture is achieved with only one more extra throw than with comparably sized, uncoated Polybutester sutures.

Surgipro II™

Surgipro II is basically a polypropylene suture which has been developed with increased resistance to fraying during knot run down especially with smaller diameters. This suture retains its tensile strength for 2 years in tissue and is extremely inert. It has a lower drag coefficient in tissue in comparison to Nylon thus making it ideal for continuous suture closure.

TIPS FOR PRESERVATION OF TENSILE STRENGTH OF SUTURE

Absorbable Sutures

1. Protect them from heat and moisture. Store them at room temperature. Avoid storage in hot areas, e.g. near steam pipes, and in sterilizers.
2. Do not soak absorbable sutures.
3. To restore pliability surgical gut can be dipped in water at room temperature or saline.
4. Synthetic absorbable sutures must be kept dry.

Nonabsorbable Sutures

1. *Silk*: Store silk in dry environment. Dry strands are stronger than wet strands. Wet silk looses up to 20% of its strength. Avoid kinking, nicking or instrument damage.
2. *Polyester fibre*: It is unaffected by moisture. It can be used either wet or dry. Handle it carefully to avoid abrasions, kinking, and nicking or instrument damage.
3. *Nylon*: Straighten kinks or bends by passing strands between gloved fingers a few times. Avoid kinking, nicking or instrument damage.
4. *Polypropylene*: Unaffected by moisture. It can be used wet or dry. Thread should be straightened with a gentle, steady and even pull.

SURGICAL NEEDLES

Composition

Surgical needles are made up of stainless steel alloy, which is resistant to corrosion and contain a minimum of 12% chromium. When a needle is exposed to oxygen in air it forms a thin protective layer of chromium oxide.

An ideal needle should have following characteristics:

1. Made of high quality stainless steel.
2. As thin and slim as possible without compromising strength.
3. Should have a stable grasp in needle holder.
4. Should cause minimal trauma to tissue.
5. Should be able to penetrate tissue with minimal resistance.
6. Should resist bending.
7. Should be resistant to breaking under a given amount of bending. An ideal needle should bend before breaking if excessive force is applied.

The Anatomy of the Needle

Components

Every surgical needle has three basic parts swage, body and point.

Swage

The swage is the site of attachment of the suture to the needle. It is usually round in section. Swaged needles produce smaller holes in tissue in comparison to threaded eye needles.

Body

The body of the needle is the portion which is grasped by the needle holder during the surgical procedure. It is often *square* in section. The diameter of the body of the needle should be as close as possible to the diameter of the suture material to minimize bleeding and leakage. This is especially important for cardiovascular, gastrointestinal and bladder procedures.

Point

The needle point extends from tip of the needle to the level of the maximum cross section of the body.

Types of Needle Point

Cutting needles have two opposing cutting edges.

Conventional Cutting Edge Needle

This has two opposite cutting edges and a third cutting edge is on the inside of the concave curvature of the needle. The inside cutting edge produces linear cuts perpendicular and near to the incision. When the suture exerts a wound closure force, it can cut through this hole. It is primarily used for closure of skin and sternum.

Reverse Cutting Edge Needle

This has a third cutting edge on the outer convex curvature of needle. It has more strength than a conventional cutting needle. The danger of tissue cut out is much less because the hole produced by it has a wide wall of the tissue contrary to the linear cut produced by a conventional cutting needle. The wide wall against which the suture is tied prevents suture cut through.

Spatula Needle

This is a side cutting needle, flat on both bottom and top, with cutting edges on the side. It is primarily used for eye surgery. It can also be used for repairing lacerations of the nail matrix. Side cutting edges split or separate the tissue without cutting them. These allow maximum ease of penetration and control as they pass between and through tissue layers.

Taper Point Needle

This tapers to a sharp tip. It spreads the tissue without cutting it, and is used where the surgeon wants to make a smallest hole possible without cutting tissue. It is used in soft tissue, e.g. vessels, abdominal viscera and fascia which do not resist needle penetration.

Taper Cut Needle

This combines the unique features of taper point and cutting edge needles. Cutting edges extends only for a short distance from the needle tip and blends in to a round taper body. The taper cut needle is used for anastomosis of calcified and fibrotic blood vessels, to graft, and for closure of defects in oral mucosa. The penetrating point needle is a type of taper cut needle with a diamond shaped point.

Blunt Point Needle

This has a taper body with a rounded, blunt point that will not cut through tissue. It is used for suturing the liver and kidney, and also to prevent needle stick injury in patients with HIV, or hepatitis B/C infection.

TYPES OF NEEDLES ACCORDING TO SHAPE

1. Straight needle: This can be used for suturing easily accessible tissue, where direct manipulation can easily be performed by the fingers (Fig. 5.1).

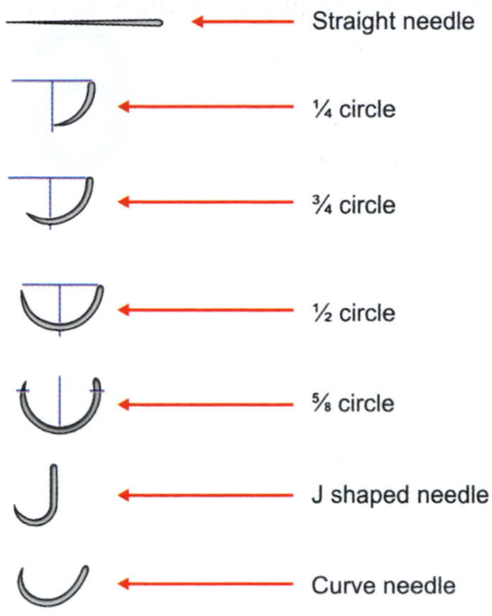

Figure 5.1: Different shapes of surgical needles

2. The Keith needle is a straight cutting needle for skin closure of abdominal wounds and for arthroscopic suturing of the meniscus in the knee.
3. Bunnell needle (BN) is used for tendon repair.
4. The half curved needle or "Ski" needle is used for laparoscopic anastomosis.
5. Curved needle: These needles have predictable needle turn out from tissue. They require less space for manoeuvring than a straight needle but require a needle holder for manipulation. The curvature of the needle may be 1/4, 3/8, 1/2, or 5/8 of a full circle. 3/8 circle is used for large superficial wounds. The curve of the needle can be manipulated with slight pronation but then has a larger arc of manipulation, so is not suitable in a deep body cavity or restricted area. 1/2 circle needle is used in a confined space. 5/8 circle needle is used for haemorrhoidectomy, in the nasal cavity, oral cavity and pelvis (Fig. 5.1).

Key Points

1. Ideal sutures having all the desirable properties do not exist.
2. One should choose a suture carefully, keeping in mind the type of operation being performed.
3. Tensile strength of suture and ease of knotting is an important aspect to be considered while selecting suture material.
4. If selecting a nonabsorbable suture one should choose a suture which maintains its tensile strength for 90–120 days, i.e. the time required for healing.
5. Surgical silk looses tensile strength when exposed to moisture.
6. Monofilament sutures are preferred for vascular surgery because of minimal tissue drag and resistance against harbouring organisms.
7. Multifilament sutures have more tensile strength, pliability, flexibility and are well suited for intestinal anastomosis.

Patient Positioning during Surgery

6

Sudhir Kumar Jain, David L Stoker

Proper positioning of the patient during surgery is of paramount importance for the proper exposure of the operative field. Poor positioning leads to poor access and increases the risk of complications in both the operative and postoperative period like pressure area damage, and nerve injuries. In this chapter, positioning of patients during common surgical procedures has been described. It is the responsibility of the surgical team to ensure that the patient's position on the table is correct. No part of the patient's body should be in contact with a metal surface if electrocautery is to be used, to avoid leaking of current from the point of contact. Excessive abduction of the upper limbs or pressure over bony prominences should be avoided to prevent neuropraxia or skin damage.

SUPINE POSITION FOR LAPAROTOMY

This is the most common position during abdominal surgery. In this position the head is padded and stabilized with various positioning aids, e.g. closed head ring or gel head cushion or double wedge cushion with padding under the shoulders. Purpose of this head stabilisation is to keep the cervical spine in the neutral position (awake) so that any pressure on the back of the head is avoided.

Usually in abdominal surgery, both arms are abducted to the side either in pronation or supination. In prone position, the arms should be abducted to approximately 60°, flexed at the elbows, and fixed with the arm positioning device. Support with a short armrest, should always be provided for the lower arm and hand. This positioning of the arm prevents wrist drop. In case abduction of the arm is required between 60° and 90°, the patient arm should be adjusted to supine position (Texas position). A pad is placed under the wrist in this position to keep nerves in the elbow free of pressure. The shoulder elevation from the level of the table enlarges the gap between clavicle and the first rib and reduces the risk of compressing the nerves. The arm must be elevated over the level of the shoulder.

The rule of thumb for positioning the arm in supine position is to elevate the shoulder from the level of the table and keep the distal joint higher than the proximal joint. So the elbow is higher than the shoulder and the wrist higher than the elbow.

Hips and knees should be preferably mildly flexed with pads placed under the lumbar spine. The pads can be in the from of a small rolled/folded towel. If necessary, a half rolled towel is placed under the knees at the distal thigh. Pressure on the heels should be reduced to a minimum. One of the methods for this can be the use of small gel mats placed under the lower leg.

NECK SURGERY

Thyroid Surgery

Patient is placed supine with the table tilted up at an angle of 15° at the head end to reduce venous engorgement. A ring is placed underneath the occipital region to stabilise the head. The neck is extended by placing a sand bag transversely across the shoulders. Neck extension makes thyroid gland, skin, platysma and strap muscles more prominent and facilitates dissection. Precautions should be taken in elderly patients and in patients with pathology of the cervical spine, and hyperextension of neck should be avoided in these cases during positioning.

Parotid Surgery

Position of the patient is supine with head resting on a ring and turned away from the side of the pathology.

POSTEROLATERAL THORACOTOMY (FIG. 6.1)

Patient is turned on the unaffected side in the lateral decubitus position with the hips secured to table by means of wide adhesive tapes. The lower leg is flexed at the knee with a pillow between the upper and lower legs. The upper leg is extended. The shoulder and upper thorax are supported by a rolled sheet or blanket placed under the axilla. Table supports are used to maintain the position and additional strapping is used at the hip for stability. The upper arm is supported by a bracket in a position of 90° flexion. The lower arm is flexed and positioned underneath the head.

LUMBAR APPROACH FOR KIDNEY (FIGS 6.2 AND 6.3)

Patient is turned on the unaffected side in the lateral position towards the edge of the operating table. Hip and knee next to the table are fully flexed with a pillow between the two legs. Patient is maintained in this position with a back support or by strapping. To increase the space for access, the trunk should be flexed on the lower side by

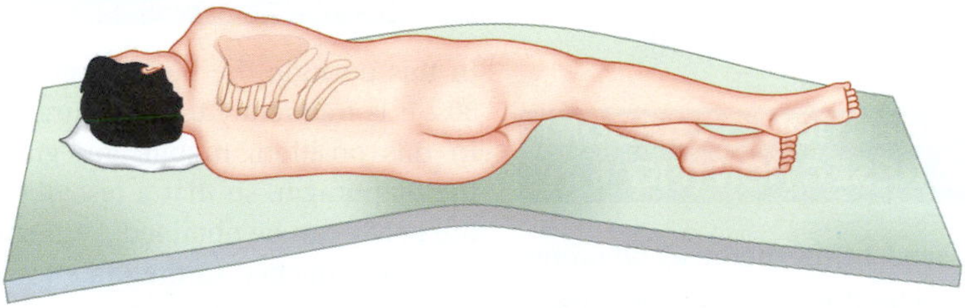

Figure 6.1: Patient position for posterolateral thoracotomy

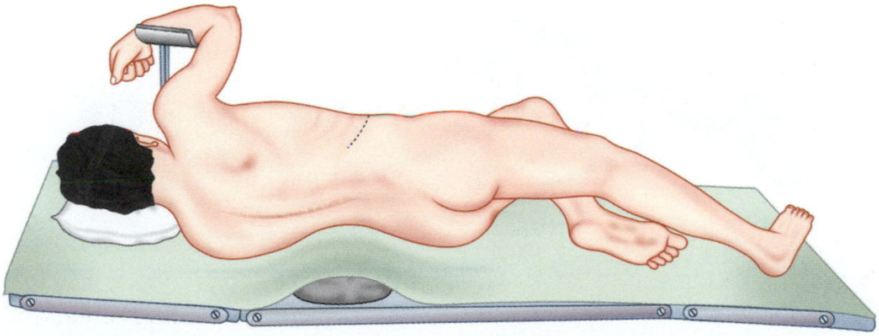

Figure 6.2: Patient position for kidney exposure

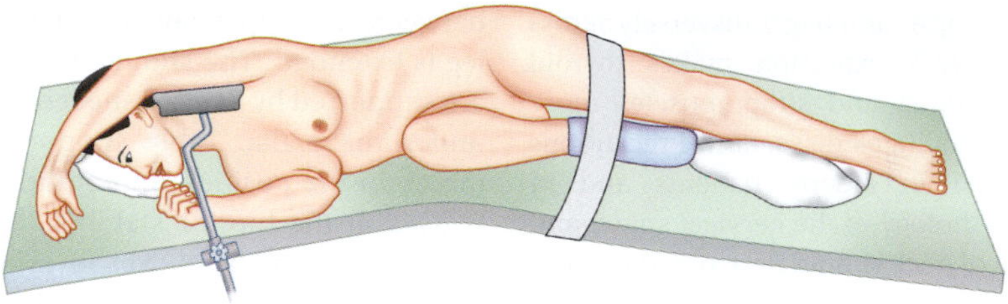

Figure 6.3: Position of patient for kidney operation through flank approach

breaking the table, or by the use of an inflatable cushion under the loin. A support for the arm prevents the shoulder from sagging forwards with consequent rotation at the waist.

MODIFIED RADICAL MASTECTOMY

The patient is placed near the edge of the operating table on the side of the surgeon. The patient lies prone with the arm and forearm on the side of the surgery outstretched on an arm board to which the wrist is secured by a bandage. The forearm is supinated so that the palm faces upwards.

ANTERIOR RESECTION OR ABDOMINOPERINEAL RESECTION (FIG. 6.4)

The patient is placed in the perineal lithotomy position with the legs in stirrups. The patient should be brought down to the edge of the table with a sand bag under the buttocks to provide proper exposure of the anal canal. The knees can be flexed but the hips should be relatively extended and the thighs abducted to allow simultaneous access to both the abdomen and the perineum. A moderate degree of head down tilt (Trendelenburg) aids in dissection.

TRENDELENBURG POSITION (FIG. 6.5)

In this position the head is tilted downwards by 30°. It is frequently used in surgery of the pelvis. In this position, mobile gut gravitates towards the diaphragm, so that a less obstructed view of the pelvis can be obtained. Well padded shoulder rests are attached to the table in such a manner that the pressure is exerted over the region of acromioclavicular region to prevent the patient

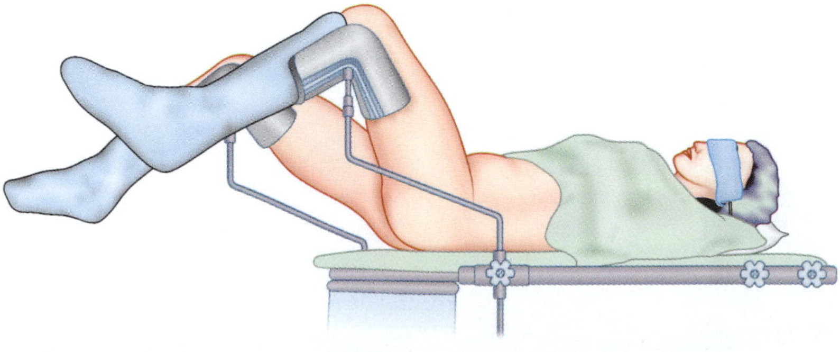

Figure 6.4: Lloyd Davis position for abdominoperineal resection

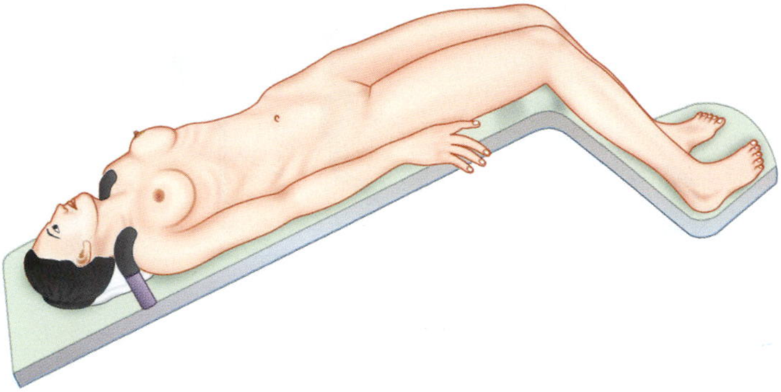

Figure 6.5: Trendelenburg position

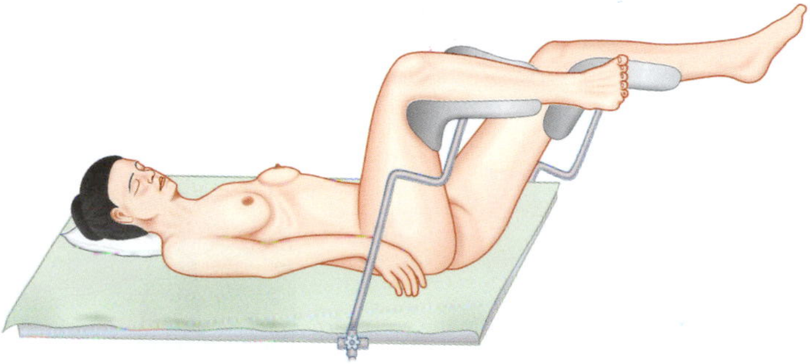

Figure 6.6: Patient position for cystoscopy

sliding head wards. If the pressure of shoulder head is applied on the root of the neck, brachial plexus injury may occur.

POSITION FOR CYSTOSCOPY (FIG. 6.6)

Patient is placed with his buttocks near the end of the table with legs abducted. The thighs should be maintained at angle of 45° with the trunk. In this position the axis of the telescope is approximately horizontal when the bladder base is being examined.

VAGINAL OPERATIONS (FIG. 6.7)

Lithotomy position is used for transvaginal procedures. In this position the patient's buttocks are on the edge of the table and rising upwards with a sandbag placed across the sacrum. The knee and hip joints are flexed at an angle of 90° with legs supported on leg rests. The thighs may be slightly abducted to generate space in between the thighs.

SURGEON'S POSITION

The operating table should be at correct height according to the operating surgeon. The surgeon should work in a comfortable and relaxed posture so that he or she does not sustain back or neck muscle strain after long hours of operating. Elbows and shoulders should be kept relaxed by the proper adjustment of height of the operating table as explained below. The surgeon should stand on the side which permits the operating hand and arm to reach the area of pathology most easily. The surgeon should stand in a position with his left foot forward and right foot back ward. In this position the surgeon's shoulder, arm and wrist are free of strain. In this position the needle is directed towards the left foot and the surgeon is

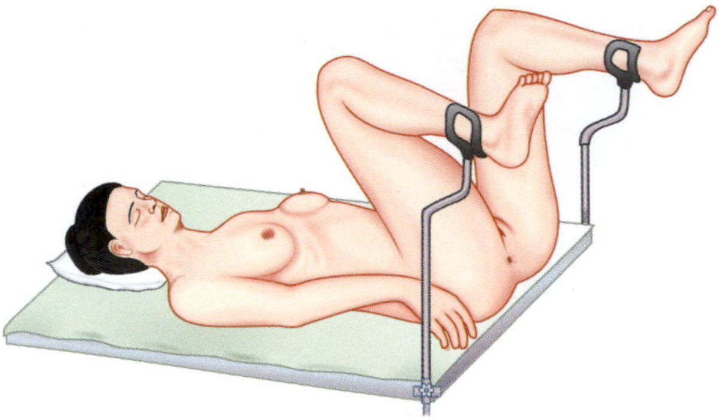

Figure 6.7: Lithotomy position for vaginal operations

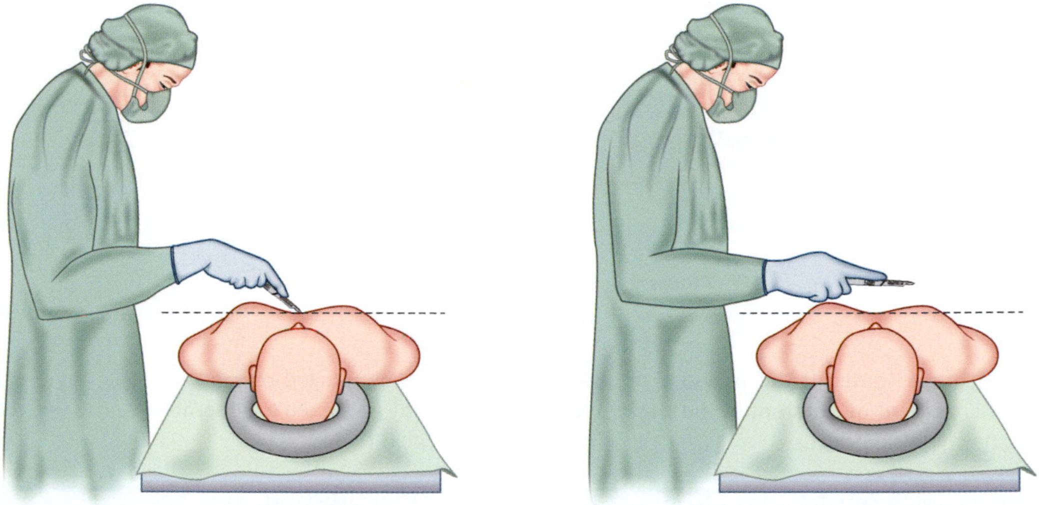

Figure 6.8: Ideal height of the operation table

able to perceive proprioceptive sensation as the needle passes through the tissue. He is able to feel the depth of tissue bites. Suturing in this position is known as forehand suturing and needs a strong biceps muscle for pronation and supination. Back hand motion is when an instrument is directed towards the right foot, and is required when cutting by scalpel or by electrocautery or during insertion of Lembert sutures.

IDEAL HEIGHT OF THE OPERATION TABLE (FIG. 6.8)

Ideal height of the operating table should be at the level of the surgeon's elbow, while operating on the abdomen or chest. If the operating table is at the level of the surgeon's elbow, the wrist is in slight dorsiflexion, which is a position of ideal function.

If the height of the operating table is higher than the level of the surgeon's elbow, there will be flexion of both elbow's and wrist. In the position of wrist flexion, long extensors of the forearm and hands will be in contraction and long flexors of the forearm and hands will be in a relaxed position, but no longer in tonic balance. This imbalance increases small muscle fatigue of the hands and reduces performance of small muscles of the hand. Eye stereopsis is more appropriate if the operating field is at a distance of 18 inches from the eyes. If the operating field is a depressed body surface, within oral cavity or within pelvis, the operating table should be below surgeon's elbow, so that the wrist is in a position of mild ulnar deviation and relatively straight. This is the functional position of the wrist, which greatly improves dexterity and strength in the fingers.

Key Points

1. Proper positioning of patient during surgery helps in the proper exposure of the operative field and facilitates the completion of a procedure with minimal stress and fatigue.
2. Improper position can complicate the surgery.
3. Avoid pressure on bony prominences.
4. Avoid excessive abduction of the upper limbs.

Anastomosis in Surgery

7

Raman Tanwar, Sudhir Kumar Jain, David L Stoker

The term 'anastomosis' is derived from a Greek word meaning 'without a mouth.' Galen (AD 131-201) was one of the earliest surgeons who used this term.

In modern day surgical practice the term anastomosis can be defined as a joining of two hollow viscera or tubular structures with an intention to restore continuity.

The need for anastomosis arises if a portion of hollow viscus has been surgically removed or destroyed by trauma, or there is a distal obstruction.

In general surgery an anastomosis may involve:

1. Gut—intestinal anastomosis.
2. Vessel—vascular anastomosis.
3. Urinary tract.
4. Biliary tract or pancreatic duct.

HISTORICAL ASPECTS

In 1826, Antoine Lembert, a French surgeon described the seromuscular suturing technique, which proved to be the mainstay of gastrointestinal surgery. Nicholas Sen from USA in 1893 described a two layered technique of intestinal anastomosis, using silk with ordinary sewing needles. Halsted, a famous surgeon described a single layer closure without incorporating the mucosa. Connell from Chicago in 1963 described an interrupted single layer technique of gut anastomosis with knots lying intraluminal and bites going through all the layers. Kocher described a two layered technique using silk and catgut. The current method of single layer extramucosal anastomosis was advocated by Matheson of Aberdeen. Alexis Carrel in 1926 described his technique of end to end vascular anastomosis which proved to be a revolution in the field of vascular surgery.

IDEAL ANASTOMOSIS

An ideal anastomotic technique should have the following features:

1. Zero leak rates.
2. Should promote early recovery of function.
3. No vascular compromise at the incised or divided margins of a viscus.
4. Should not narrow the lumen of a viscus.
5. Easy to learn, teach and perform.
6. Technique should preferably be quick to perform.

Such an ideal technique is still to emerge.

TYPES OF ANASTOMOSIS

1. End to end anastomosis.
2. End to side anastomosis.
3. Side to side anastomosis.

INTESTINAL ANASTOMOSIS

Intestinal anastomosis may involve:

1. Joining two ends of similar type of gut, i.e. jejuno-jejunal or ileo-ileal or colo-colic.

2. Joining two different types of gut, i.e. oesophagus and jejunum, stomach and jejunum, ileum and colon or rectum.
3. Joining of gut with another hollow tubular structure, e.g.
   a. Common hepatic duct and jejunum—hepaticojejunostomy.
   b. Common bile duct and duodenum—choledochoduodenostomy.
   c. Common bile duct and jejunum—choledochojejunostomy.
   d. Gallbladder and jejunum—cholecysto —jejunostomy.
   e. Pancreatic duct and jejunum—pancreaticojejunostomy.
   f. Ureters may be implanted into an ileal conduit or in to the sigmoid colon.

Vascular Anastomosis

Vascular anastomosis may involve the aorta, a peripheral artery or vein, coronary arteries or cerebral arteries.

Techniques of Anastomosis

Anastomosis can be:

1. Hand sewn using sutures.
2. Stapled.
3. Sutureless anastomosis using laser (Nd:YAG) or tissue glue, e.g. fibrin glue. These are still experimental. Fibrin glue has been used to reinforce anastomotic suture lines.

Factors which Increase the Rate of Anastomotic Leak

Emergency surgery, if associated with a hypovolemic condition, as in abdominal trauma with intra-abdominal bleeding. Hypovolemia compromises the splanchnic circulation, which may result in ischemia at the site of anastomosis.

Peritonitis is a major risk factor. Most patients with peritonitis have septicemia with a systemic inflammatory response syndrome (SIRS). Here, there are high circulating levels of inflammatory mediators, which induce excessive inflammation, (more than required for wound healing) at the site of anastomosis, rendering it friable and prone to leak.

Low hemoglobin concentration may cause decreased oxygen carrying capacity of the blood, inducing relative ischemia at the site of anastomosis.

Malnutrition leads to low levels of serum protein and albumin, causing interstitial tissue edema, increased suture tension, and poor healing.

Previous irradiation: Patients who have been irradiated for malignancy have a higher incidence of anastomotic leak because irradiation induces fibrosis and reduces blood supply.

Immunosuppressive drugs including steroids cause poor tissue healing.

Unprepared gut: An anastomosis performed on unprepared colon with a high fecal bacterial load has an increased chance of leak.

Malignancy, infection and inflammation will all impair healing.

Distal obstruction should be excluded before joining two ends. Ongoing obstruction will lead to increased tissue tension and ischemia.

Ongoing tension on an anastomosis may be seen due to mechanical twists, and may also occur secondary to a narrow lumen, not wide enough to allow passage of fluid. This also leads to ischemia, and the possibility of anastomotic dehiscence.

The Hand Sewn Anastomosis: Technical Issues (Figs 7.1 and 7.2)

Choice of Suture Material

One should choose a suture material which induces the least inflammatory reaction. Majority of sutures available today act as a foreign body and induce inflammation. It has been seen that silk induces a significantly greater cellular reaction at the site of anastomosis, which persists up to 6 weeks in comparison to Polypropylene, Polyglycolic acid or Polyglactin. An ideal suture material for anastomosis should cause minimal inflammation and tissue reaction and should provide maximum strength during the lag phase of wound healing. Monofilament and coated braided sutures are most effective but still not ideal.

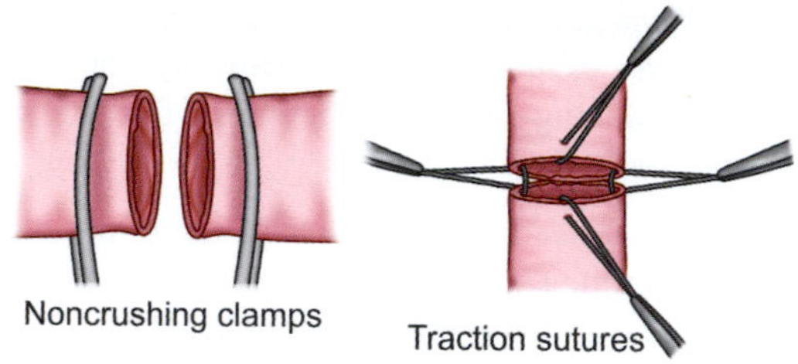

Figure 7.1: Preparation of gut to form an anastomosis. Noncrushing clamps are applied to prevent leakage and ends are held together by traction sutures

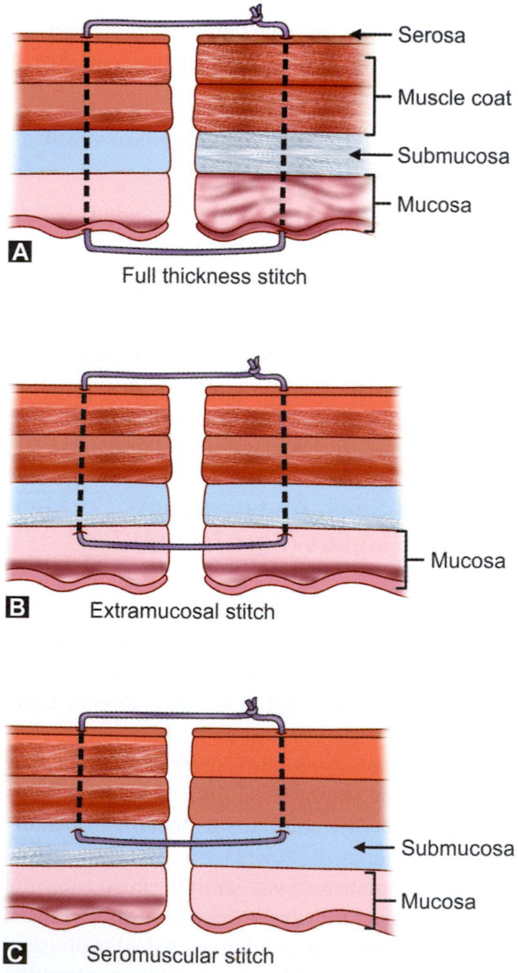

Figures 7.2A to C: (A) Full thickness stitch (above); (B) Extramucosal stitch; and (C) Seromuscular stitch

Continuous versus Interrupted Sutures (Figs 7.3 and 7.4)

Till date no randomised trial has established the superiority of one technique over the other but in experimental studies using rat model, perianastomotic oxygen tension was found to be lower with continuous sutures. Narrowing of the lumen may occur with continuous sutures especially in the early phase when postoperative edema tends to tighten the suture. There may sometimes be a drawstring effect also.

Single Layer versus Double Layer Anastomosis

Double layer anastomosis which came into vogue before single layer anastomosis was traditionally thought to be more secure. However, studies have clearly shown the advantages of single layer anastomosis in the form of decreased operative time, less narrowing of intestinal lumen, more rapid vascularisation and mucosal healing, rapid increase in the strength of the anastomosis in the first few postoperative days and the early postoperative return of normal bowel function as measured by return of bowel sounds, passage of flatus and resumption of oral feeding.

Types of Sutured Anastomosis

There are multiple techniques in use, but the authors have described only those techniques which are in common use and widely accepted. One should adopt one of these techniques and try to master it.

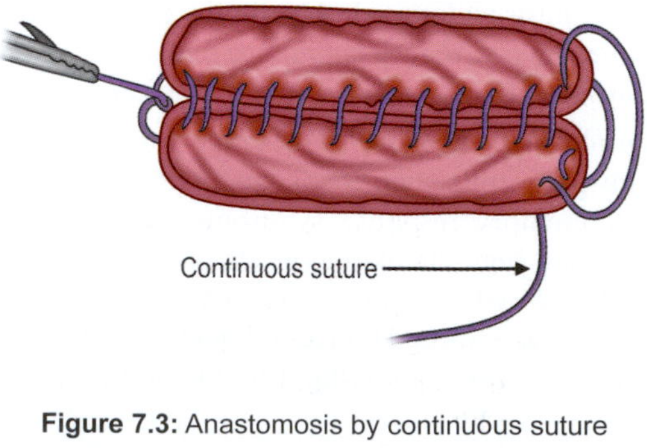

Figure 7.3: Anastomosis by continuous suture

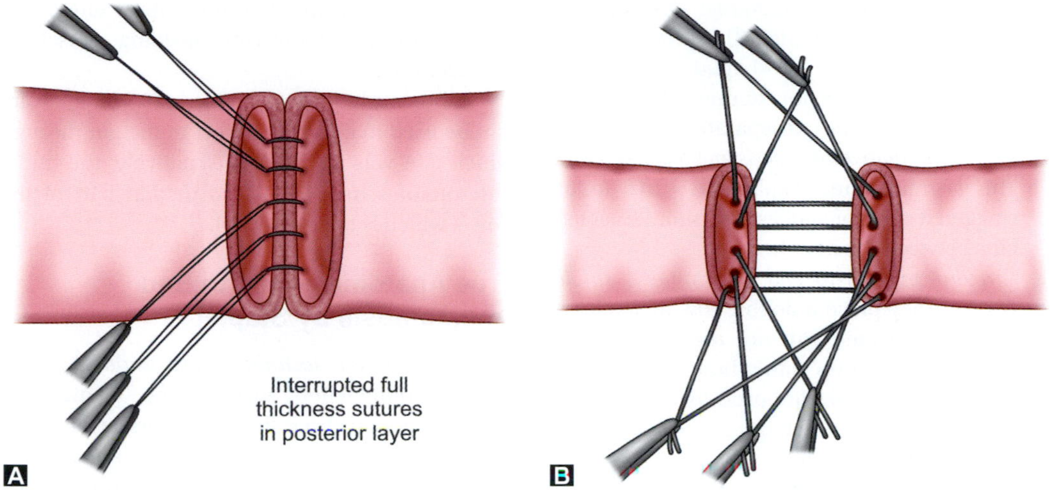

Figures 7.4A and B: (A) Method of anastomosis of bowel if the ends are fixed. Posterior layer stitches are applied first; (B) If one of the ends is mobile, stitches are left with ends separated until all posterior wall sutures have been inserted. Mobile end can be railroaded along the sutures and the knots tied. This is also known as the 'telescoping' technique

The Single Layer Anastomosis

There are three types:

1. A single layer interrupted extramucosal technique is preferred by many. This is mainly used for large or small bowel anastomosis.
2. Single layer interrupted full thickness. This is mainly used in biliary surgery, e.g. hepaticojejunostomy and choledochoduodenostomy.
3. Single layer full thickness continuous technique is commonly employed for gastrojejunal anastomosis. The continuous suture gives the advantage of hemostasis, as the gastric wall is very vascular. It also reduces intraoperative time.

The Two Layer Anastomosis

The two layered anastomosis consists of an inner layer taking a bite through the full thickness of the viscus. This inner layer can be continuous or interrupted depending upon the portion of the viscus to be anastomosed. For small bowel, the inner layer can be continuous, but for colon the inner layer can be interrupted or continuous depending on the surgeon's choice. The outer layer takes a bite through the seromuscular layer only and is usually interrupted in colonic surgery. In small bowel or stomach it is usually continuous.

The Stapled Anastomosis

Surgical stapling devices were first introduced by Hulti in 1908 but did not gain popularity because the instruments were cumbersome, unreliable and difficult to use. The past three decades have seen the development of reliable, disposable surgical stapling devices which produce consistent quality staple lines with rare technical failures. With the help of these stapling devices anastomosis at difficult sites such as low rectum, or high esophagus has become safer and more technically feasible. The drawbacks of stapling devices are that they are costly and the surgeon is as much reliant on technology as on his surgical skills. The main advantage of these devices is that they save time and may have a place where multiple anastomosis have to be created, e.g. in Whipple's procedure, or in radical cystectomy with ileal conduit reconstruction.

Staplers

Three types of staplers are in vogue for creating intestinal anastomosis.

1. *Transverse anastomosis stapler (TA)*: It is the simplest type of stapler. This device places two staggered rows of B shaped staples across the bowel but does not cut them. The surgeon needs to divide the gut separately.
2. *Gastrointestinal anastomosis linear cutter (GIA)*: This gastrointestinal stapler places two double staggered rows of staples and simultaneously cuts between the double rows.
3. *Circular or end to end anastomosis stapler (EEA)*: They place a double row of staples in a circle and then cuts out the tissue within the circle of staples with a built in cylindrical knife. These staples are used for low anterior resection, gastroesophageal anastomosis or for stapled hemorrhoidopexy.

There is also an Endo GIA gun which is used for laparoscopic surgery. Staples are made up of titanium, which causes little tissue reaction, and is non magnetic, thus enabling future MRI scanning. Staplers can produce:

1. Functional end to end anastomosis.
2. Anatomical end to end anastomosis.
3. Side to side anastomosis.

Functional Stapled End to End Anastomosis

The steps of a functional end to end anastomosis are:

1. Place two cut ends of the bowel side to side, maintaining the orientation of mesentery.
2. Insert the two limbs of GIA stapler, one each in to lumen of either bowel ends either through an enterotomy or through the open end of the bowel. Engage the two limbs of the stapler in to each other, making sure that the mesentery of the gut does not get caught in the staple line. This can be ensured by putting a finger in between the mesenteries when the stapler is engaged.
3. The stapler is then fired to fuse the two bowel walls into a single septum and to create a cut between the two rows of staples.
4. Wait for one minute before removing the stapler for the hemostasis to occur (This is not always necessary but is a useful precaution).
5. Inspect the staple line for completeness and hemostasis. Under-run bleeding vessels if necessary.

A noncutting linear stapler (TA) or a suture can be used to close the defect in the gut through which GIA was inserted. Alternatively, the initial enterotomies may be placed in that part of the bowel which is to be resected.

True Anatomical End to End Anastomosis by Stapler

1. *Triangulation technique*: Cut ends of bowel are triangulated together by taking stay sutures and three linear staplers are fired in intersecting vectors to achieve a complete closure. Drawback of this technique is that staple lines are everted (Figs 7.5A to D).
2. Two cut ends of the bowel can be united together by using an EEA stapler, which produces a directly apposed, inverted stapled end to end anastomosis. This is not used much now as more often end to side technique is used.

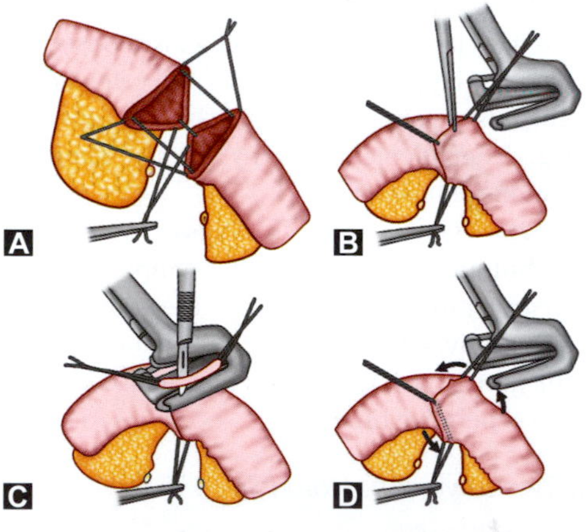

Figures 7.5A to D: Showing triangulation technique of end to end anastomosis by stapler: (A) Three stay sutures at three corners of divided ends of gut to triangulate the ends; (B) Linear staplers applied between two stay sutures; (C)Excess tissue above staple line excised; (D) Gut rotated and similar process repeated between remaining stay sutures

Advantages of Stapled Anastomosis over Hand Sewn Anastomosis

1. Titanium staples used in anastomosis provoke minimal inflammatory response.
2. They provide support to the cut surfaces in lag phase (weakest phase of healing).
3. Stapling may shorten operating time especially in low pelvic anastomosis, or in the thorax, or high abdomen.
4. After resection of tumour, recurrence at the staple line is much less than at the suture line because suture materials produce a more pronounced cellular proliferation than staples.
5. Stapled anastomosis heal by primary intention but sutured anastomosis heal by secondary intention.

Inverted Suture Line versus Everted Suture Line

An inverted suture line is found to be better than an everted suture line in terms of bursting pressure, rate of healing and degree of inflammation. An inverted suture line has a greater aesthetic appeal although this has little relevance to healing.

Testing the Anastomosis

In certain situations where an anastomosis is performed in a difficult situation, e.g. low anorectal anastomosis, esophagogastric anastomosis or where the anastomosis is complex as in the creation of an ileoanal pouch, testing of anastomosis is important. Anastomosis can be tested by following methods:

The Underwater Test

This test is performed in cases of low anterior resection (LAR) or in cases of esophagogastric anastomosis. A soft noncrushing clamp is applied on gastric side or on the sigmoid colon just distal to the anastomosis. Pelvic cavity or left subdiaphragmatic space is filled with saline. Air is insufflated from the anal opening in case of LAR or nasogastric tube in case of esophagogastric anastomosis. If there is no bubbling of air into the saline the anastomosis is airtight, and presumed to be safe.

The Methylene Blue Test

This test is performed in cases of gastric pouch surgery for obesity. After completion of the anastomosis, methylene blue is injected through a nasogastric tube. There should not be any leak of methylene blue from the gastrojejunostomy.

Protecting an Anastomosis

Nasogastric Decompression

Routine nasogastric decompression is not mandatory after lower intestinal anastomosis unless there is a significant paralytic ileus with abdominal distension, gastric dilatation or excessive emesis.

In upper gastrointestinal anastomosis, e.g. gastrojejunostomy or gastroduodenal anastomosis nasogastric suction is essential for 3–5 days to avoid any tension on the suture line caused by retention of gastric secretions. Gastric motility takes around 72 hours to recover and a nasogastric tube may prevent acute gastric dilatation. Stents are left across anastomosis following hepaticojejunostomy and pancreaticojejunostomy to prevent bile or pancreatic leaks. A nasogastric tube is left after every emergency laparotomy. An unwanted side effect of nasogastric tube placement is discomfort in the pharynx, and difficulty in coughing, along with increased risk of upper airway tract infection.

Abdominal Drains after Intestinal Anastomosis

The ability of abdominal drainage to "protect" an anastomosis has been challenged by Yates. The peritoneal cavity cannot be drained effectively by a single drain due to the rapid development of adhesions and sealing of the drainage tract. Severe inflammatory reactions have been shown to occur around the drains. An intra-abdominal drain after anterior resection or ileo-anal anastomosis is kept in the pelvis because there is higher than usual incidence of fluid collections in the pelvis after these operations.

General Principles of Intestinal Anastomosis

1. There should not be any disparity between the two ends of lumen to be joined together. If one end is narrower than other, it can be enlarged by giving a cut along the antimesenteric border sometimes also known as "fish mouthing" of the end.
2. To prevent leakage of contents and to steady the two ends, either noncrushing clamps can be applied across the gut or stay sutures can be taken at the end.
3. Three types of suture can be used for anastomosis of the gut:
   a. All coat stitches in which bites are taken through all layers of the gut. This was advocated by William Halsted (1852–1922) (Fig. 7.2A).
   b. In extra-mucosal or sero-submucosal technique all layers are included except mucosa. Submucosa is the strongest layer, as it contains plenty of collagen tissue (Fig. 7.2B).
   c. In seromuscular stitch bites are taken through the serosa and part of the muscular layer. This was described by a surgeon from Paris (Antoine Lembert). This stitch is also known as a Lembert stitch. It is generally used as a second layer to strengthen the first layer.

BASIC ARTERIAL SURGICAL TECHNIQUES

Arterial surgery is generally undertaken to:

1. Repair arteries after trauma
2. Reconstruct arteries which are diseased or blocked.

Arterial surgery like all other anastomosis should be undertaken in optimum conditions with good light, good exposure and good control of bleeding.

Precautions during Arterial Anastomosis

1. Handle arteries gently, and veins with extreme gentleness.
2. Vessels should be held by the adventitial tissue whenever possible to avoid trauma to the vessel wall.
3. If one needs to handle the arterial wall directly, use the tip of closed dissecting forceps.
4. Use a suture which passes easily without causing trauma and which causes least tissue reaction. A monofilament suture such as Prolene is an excellent choice.
5. Round bodied needles are used for the majority of vessels but taper cut needles are better for dense graft material or for heavily diseased arteries.
6. The needle should be passed from inside outwards—from intima to adventitia. This pins down atherosclerotic plaques to prevent the formation of intimal flaps which may lead to dissection, embolization or thrombosis.
7. Suture material should not be held with dissecting forceps, needle holders or forceps, all of which can damage the thread.
8. Knots should be hand tied.
9. When a needle has to be passed from adventitia to intima (from outside to inside) the intima should be supported against the vessel wall as the needle is inserted.
10. The needle should pass at right angles to the arterial wall and should be passed through the wall along the arc of the needle without deploying excessive force, to avoid splitting or tearing the delicate vessel wall.
11. The suture line should be smooth and everted. This provides good intimal apposition and prevents platelet aggregation on the suture line.
12. When suturing a transverse defect in an artery, start from the outside in on the upstream side and from inside out on the downstream side, in order to avoid dissection of intima from the arterial wall by turbulent blood flow. This technique helps in preventing a dissecting aneurysm especially in the aorta.

13. Vascular sutures may be:
    a. *Unlocked continuous*: Continuous unlocked sutures form a spiral around the artery, which tightens with each distending pulsation of the vessel. A tightened spiral reduces the likelihood of leakage. If a continuous suture is locked, the spiral effect will be lost and the suture will not become tightened with arterial pulsations.
    b. *Interrupted sutures*: These are used for small vessels to reduce the risk of stenosis. They are also used in children, to permit the growth of vessel circumference along with the growth of child. A draw back of interrupted sutures is increased risk of bleeding when the sutures separate with distension of vessels.
    c. *Mattress sutures*: Mattress sutures are not generally used in vascular surgery because they tend to narrow the lumen. Sometimes a single mattress suture may be used to initiate eversion or in case of diseased arteries when there is danger of simple sutures cutting out.

The Arteriotomy (Fig. 7.6)

An arteriotomy should be longitudinal to permit visualisation of the vessel lumen and to permit approaches to branches of the artery. In cases of vessels less than 4 mm in diameter, where an arteriotomy has been made only for embolectomy, a transverse incision can be made which has the advantage of less narrowing of the lumen. Closure of an arteriotomy is performed by a continuous unlocking suture with intimal apposition and eversion of cut edges. The nonintimal layer of the arterial wall should not come in contact with flowing blood unless an endarterectomy has been performed. As it may be difficult to include all layers in the suture at the end of the arteriotomy, two appropriately sized double ended arterial sutures are used. Closure is started from either end with both needles passing from inside out. Sutures are tied and secured in a pair of rubber shod forceps.

Suturing is continued from both ends using fine, evenly spaced stitches, until one reaches the apex of the vessel. The two sutures from both ends are then tied at the apex.

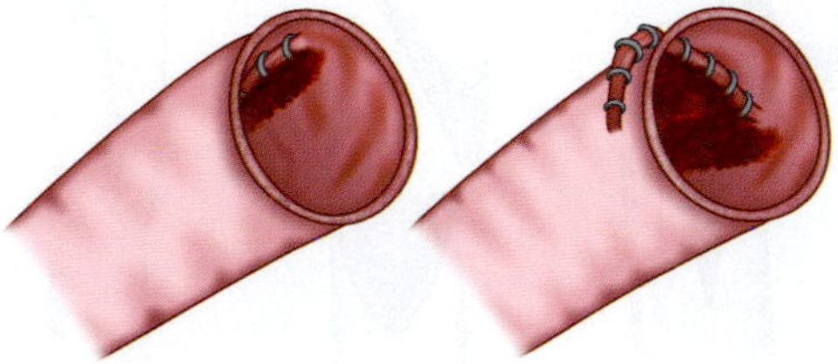

Figure 7.6: Arteriotomy in a small size vessel should be longitudinal, because clot if formed on suture line will cause less narrowing of lumen if formed around longitudinal suture line in comparison to a transverse suture line

Vein Patch Graft

Vein patch grafts are used to close an arteriotomy if it is likely that simple closure will result in narrowing of the lumen of the artery. The chances of narrowing after simple closure of an arteriotomy are greater if the artery is smaller than the diameter of the common femoral artery or if the closure of a diseased segment of artery is performed. Vein patches are usually from autologous long saphenous vein taken from the ankle or from one of the groin tributaries. Proximal long saphenous vein should not be sacrificed as it may be utilized for future vascular reconstructive procedures. If suitable vein is not available then a patch of Dacron or expanded polytetrafluoroethylene (e-PTFE) can be used.

Steps of Arteriotomy Closure Using Vein Patch Graft (Fig. 7.7)

1. A suitable vein patch graft or synthetic graft patch is prepared by trimming one end to form an ellipse that will fit into the end of the incision. Do not cut the other end, because the excess portion can be used to handle the patch without damaging the intima.
2. Take a suitable size double needled Prolene suture on a round bodied needle. Insert both needles from outside in, at one end of the vein patch. Pass needles from inside to outside through one cut end of the incision in the artery in such a manner that the suture is

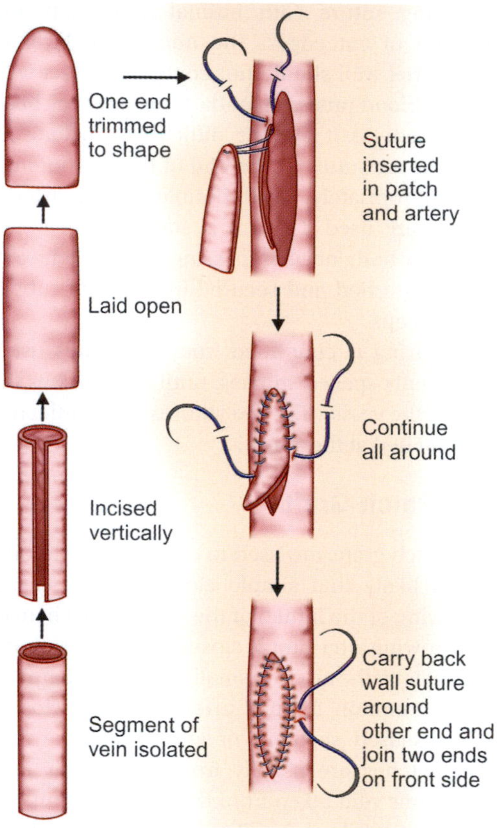

Figure 7.7: Steps of vein patch insertion to close an arteriotomy

divided into two halves to cover each side of the incision.

3. Continue taking continuous over and over sutures on the back wall and front wall using one needle each.
4. Once the half way point is reached, trim the end of the vein patch to a rounded ellipse to fit in the remaining defect. While trimming the other end of vein patch, make sure that tension on the suture is not loosened.
5. After trimming the vein patch, continue suturing on such that suture from one side is carried back around the other end and two ends of suture are tied at the mid point of the front side.

End to End Anastomosis (Figs 7.8 and 7.9)

General Principles

1. Bevel the ends of the arteries to be united to avoid narrowing except in large vessels. Bevelling can be done by cutting the ends obliquely.
2. Use continuous unlocked sutures except in children to avoid hampering of growth and in very small or delicate vessels.

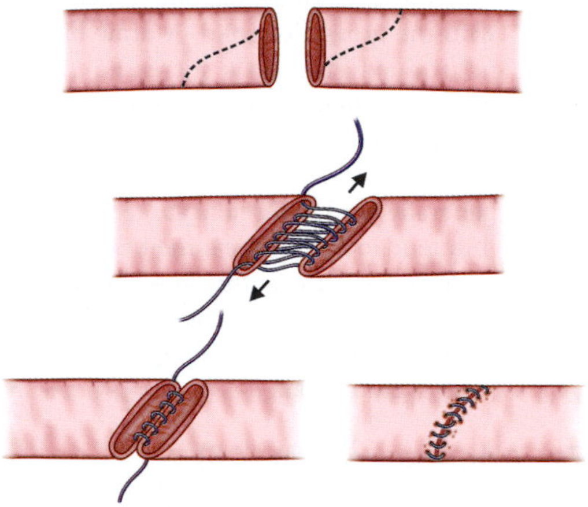

Figure 7.8: Method of performing end to end arterial anastomosis. Ends are bevelled by cutting obliquely before performing anastomosis to prevent narrowing

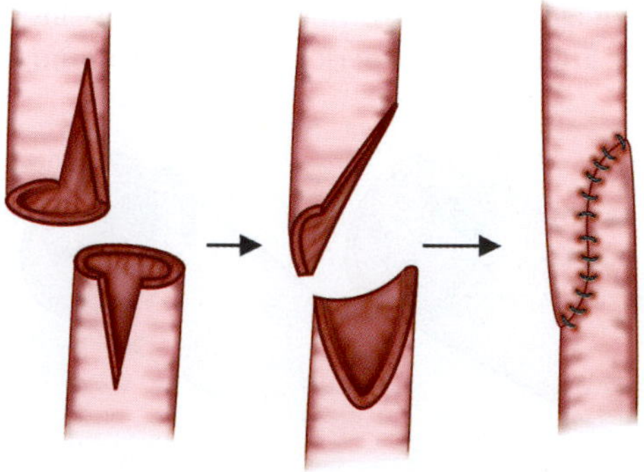

Figure 7.9: End to end arterial anastomosis. Ends are bevelled to avoid narrowing

3. Pediatric vessels are more prone to go in to spasm, so handle them gently.
4. Place sutures from outside to inside on the upstream side and from inside to outside on down stream side. There are two techniques of performing vascular anastomosis:
   a. *Anchoring suture technique*: First the anchoring sutures are placed and then the vessel is rotated, so that all sutures are placed from outside.
   b. *Parachuting technique.*

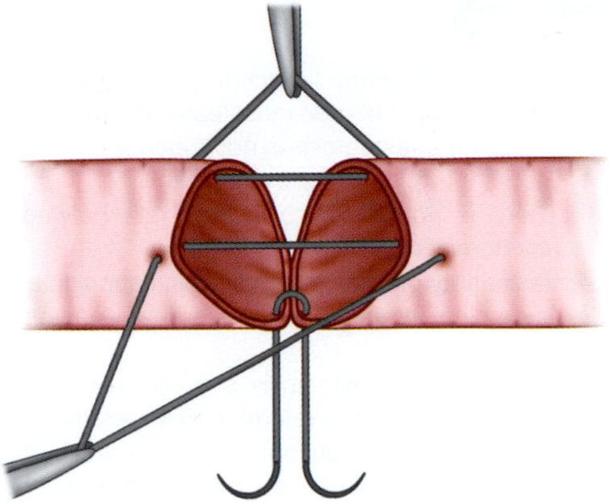

Figure 7.10: Anchoring suture technique for vascular anastomosis

Anchoring Suture Technique (Fig. 7.10)

Three anchoring sutures are placed at equal distance around the whole circumference of the vessels. These sutures are used for rotating the vessel for the purpose of gaining access. This technique is very good where mobility of vessels is not restricted.

Parachuting Technique (Fig. 7.11)

This is useful if the mobility of vessels is restricted by branches. In this technique the vessels are kept apart. A posterior row of continuous unlocked sutures is applied first using a double needled suture starting from the posterior midline and working outwards alternatively on each side, continuing around upto the front. Ends of the vessels are then gently drawn or parachuted together. Parachuting is only possible if a frictionless polypropylene suture is used.

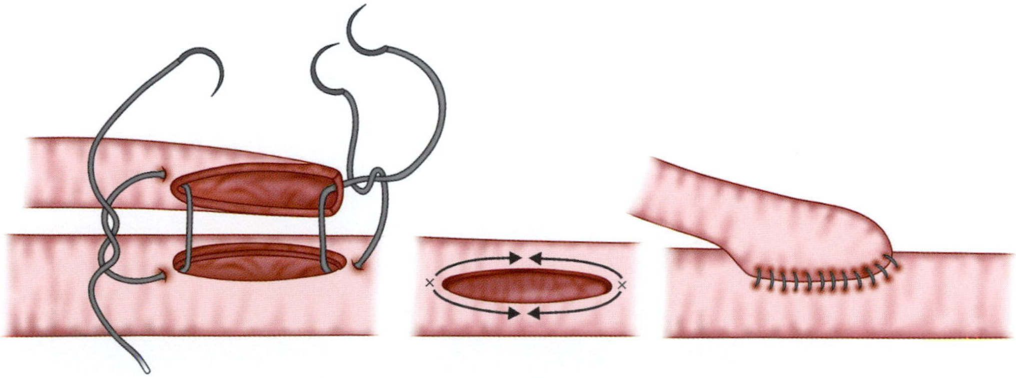

Figure 7.11: Parachuting technique

Key Points

1. The ideal anastomotic technique is still to emerge.
2. Every surgical trainee must learn and master hand sewn anastomotic techniques.
3. A stapled anastomosis is not superior to a hand sewn one, but it may save time.
4. Staplers add to the cost of surgery.
5. There is no difference in leak rate between continuous and interrupted sutures following intestinal anastomosis.
6. Vascularity of resected ends of gut should be ensured before joining them.
7. Abdominal drainage after intestinal anastomosis should be avoided except in cases of peritonitis or trauma.
8. Single layer anastomosis scores over double layer technique in terms of time saving, less luminal narrowing and early return of postoperative bowel function.
9. During arterial anastomosis, hold arteries by periarterial or advential tissue to avoid trauma to arterial wall.
10. Monofilament suture, i.e. prolene with round body needle is the suture of choice for arterial anastomosis.
11. For an arterial anastomosis the needle should pass from inside to outside to prevent formation of intimal flaps and to fix any atherosclerotic plaque.

Never try to load or unload the blade on to the handle by hand. This should only be attempted with the blade being held in forceps. To load the blade onto a scalpel handle, hold the blade in artery forceps near the base of cutting edge and advance it in to the scalpel, until the lower end of the blade fits into a groove on the handle and you hear a click (Fig. 8.3). To unload the blade, hold the base of the blade and then lift it up and pull it out of the groove, again using a pair of forceps (Fig. 8.4).

The scalpel can be held as a table knife for a skin incision. The knife is held at 30 degrees or less from the horizontal in a pronated hand, between the thumb and middle finger with the index finger at the base of the blade on the upper surface to apply and control pressure. Grip is strengthened by wrapping the ring and little finger around the handle, which rests on the hypothenar muscles (Fig. 8.5).

For a small, precise cut, the scalpel is held like a pen (Fig. 8.6). It is a good surgical practice to mark the incision with a skin marking pencil or with the back of the blade before actually incising it. Blade numbers 20 to 24 have a wider shaft and are used for larger incisions and dissection. Number 15 blades have a narrower shaft and are used for smaller incisions, for example when making port sites for laparoscopic surgery, or when removing small skin lesions. The number 11 blade is also known as a stab knife, and is used for incision and drainage of abscesses and to incise skin for inserting drains.

THE SCISSORS

Scissors are very useful and versatile instruments. They can be used for:

1. Tissue dissection.
2. Undermining skin or raising skin flaps.

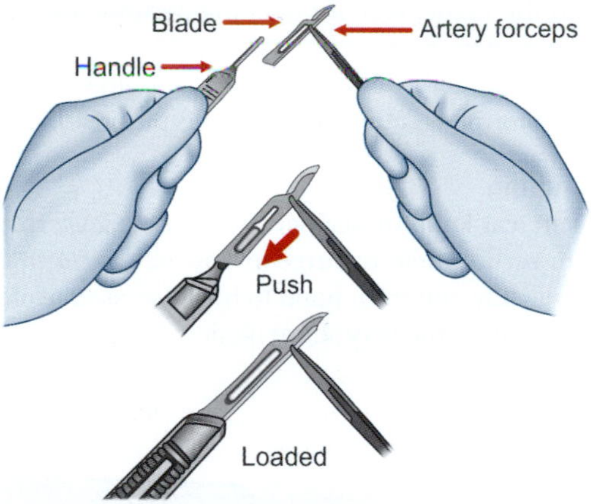

Figure 8.3: Steps for loading a blade on scalpel handle

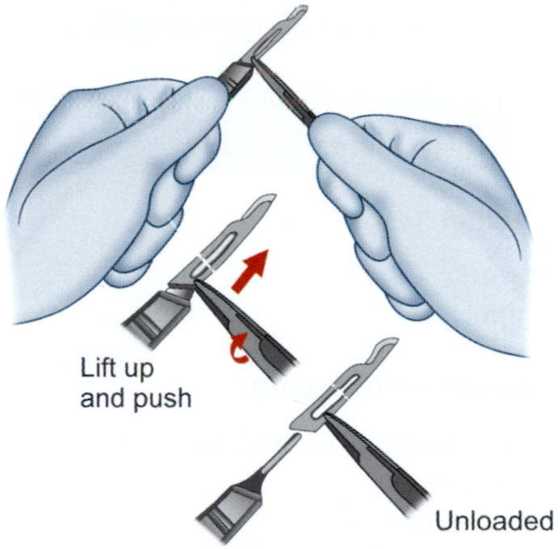

Figure 8.4: Steps for unloading a blade from a scalpel handle

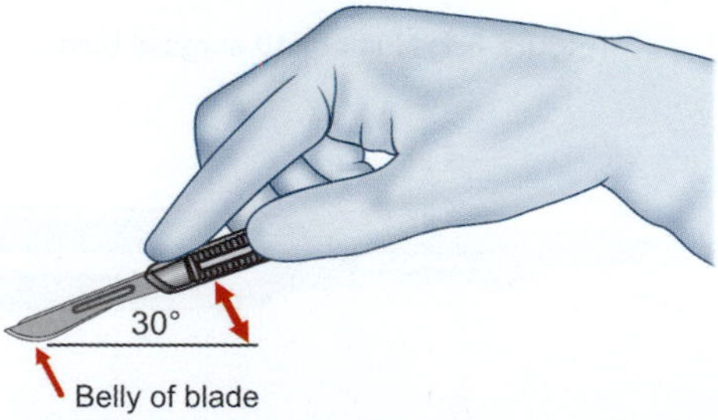

Figure 8.5: Method of holding scalpel as a table knife

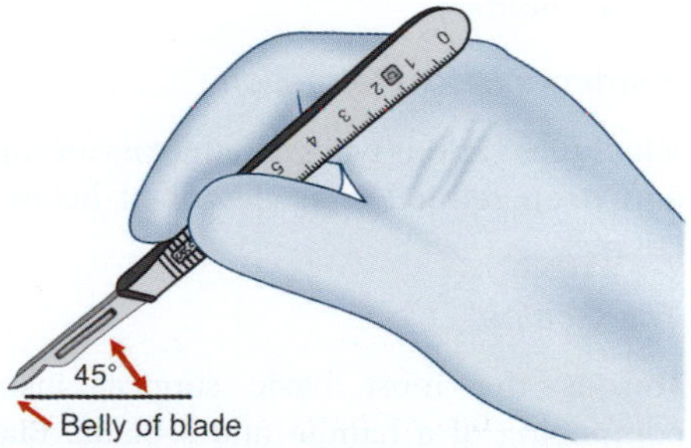

Figure 8.6: Method of holding scalpel as a pen

Art of Instrument Handling

8

Sudhir Kumar Jain, David L Stoker

INTRODUCTION

Every surgeon must learn to properly handle common instruments used in day to day surgical practice in order to avoid injury to the surgical team or the patient and to prevent malfunctioning of instruments. In this chapter, basic instrument handling techniques have been described.

BROAD CLASSIFICATION OF INSTRUMENTS

Instruments for Cutting

1. Scissors
2. Scalpel

Instruments for Grasping

1. Thumb forceps (toothed/nontoothed)
2. Artery forceps
3. Babcock forceps
4. Ellis forceps

Instrument for Suturing

Needle holders

Instruments for Retraction

It includes various types of retractors for superficial and deep retraction as described below in this chapter.

The Scalpel

This is the most basic surgical instrument, comprising of a handle and a blade. Blades are disposable and the handle is reusable. The handle is commonly known as a BP handle after Bard Parker, the inventor. It comes in two sizes 3, and 4. The number 3 handle will accommodate a small sized surgical blade from numbers 10 to 15 (Figs 8.1 and 8.2). The number 4 handle will accommodate larger blades ranging from sizes 18 to 24. Scalpel can be used for making deliberate controlled cut in to the tissue, e.g. for opening peritoneum, for making skin incision, for raising skin flaps as in thyroid surgery or mastectomy (although many surgeons use electrocautery for this purpose).

Handling

A surgical knife or scalpel should be transferred from scrub nurse to surgeon and *vice versa* in a kidney tray, not from hand to hand, so as to avoid injuries from the very sharp blade.

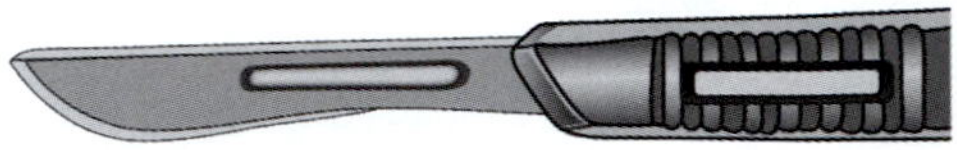

Figure 8.1: Number 10 surgical blade

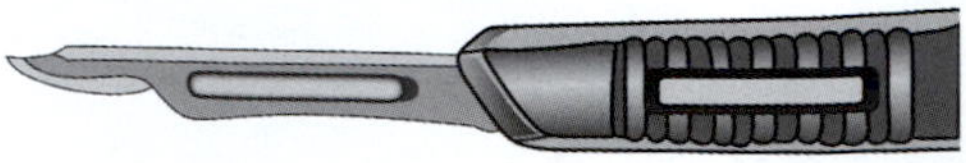

Figure 8.2: Number 15 surgical blade

3. Dividing tissue.
4. Cutting sutures.
5. Cutting gauze, meshes or other surgical materials.
6. Spreading and opening tissue planes.
7. Assisting the surgeon in the palpation of tissues.
8. Probing cavities
9. The closed scissors may be swept from side to side and used as a tissue elevator and blunt dissector.

Types of Scissors

1. Dissecting scissors with a blunt tip.
2. Cutting scissors with a sharp tip.

Scissors have two blades—one is a moving and cutting blade, while the other is stationary. Scissors can be straight or curved. Cutting scissors are known as Mayo's scissors and are used for cutting heavy fascia and sutures. Lighter dissecting scissors such as Metzenbaum or McIndoe's scissors are used for dissecting and cutting delicate tissue. They have a longer handle to blade ratio. A typical pair of scissors measure 6 inches which is designed and balanced for a normal size adult hand. Longer sized scissors are only to be used if one is working inside the depth of body cavity or in large surgical wound which requires extra, length of handle to reach the tissue. The tips of scissors can be sharp or blunt. If dissecting in dense scar tissue sharp pointed pairs of scissors are required which can penetrate the collagen bundles easily. If the surgeon is dissecting in loose tissue planes without fibrous tissue blunt tipped scissors are used which make dissection fast and safe. Scissors with curved blades gives flexibility of approach angle and makes it possible to lift and palpate tissue to greater extent in comparison to straight scissors.

Straight blade scissors are ideal for cutting ends of sutures or ligatures. Straight blade scissors allow rapid and accurate positioning of scissor tip before cutting.

Handling (Fig. 8.7)

Each blade has a ring at the end, also known as a bow. For holding scissors, the hand should be in a mid pronated position. The distal phalanx of the thumb should go into the ring of the moving blade and the distal phalanx of the ring finger into the other ring. The ring should never go beyond the distal interphalangeal joint. The tip of the index finger should rest over the joint of the blades and middle finger should wrap around the handle to steady it. While dividing tissues or sutures in a cavity, the scissor blades should rest over the index finger of the nondominant hand to steady them, and to minimise tremors.

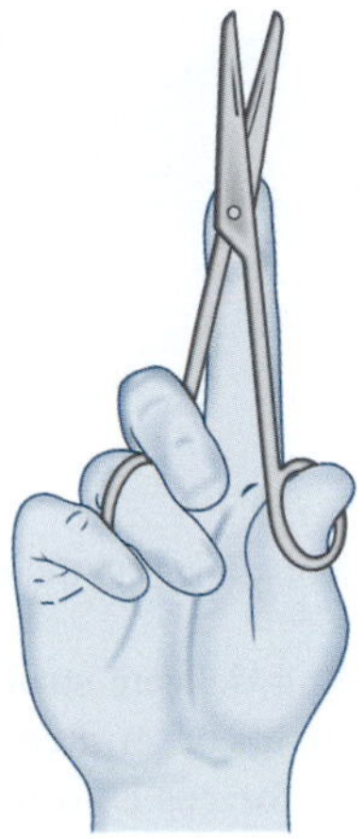

Figure 8.7: Method of holding scissors

In a vertical direction scissors cut from near to far and in a transverse direction from dominant to the nondominant side. If you want to cut from nondominant to dominant side or from far to near, it is advisable to use a scalpel unless skilled in using scissors in either hands. Some surgeons point the direction of blades towards the elbow while cutting from left to right with the right hand.

THUMB FORCEPS AND TISSUE HOLDING FORCEPS

These consist of two shafts held together at one end with a spring device that holds the shafts open. The tips of forceps can be smooth, serrated or have teeth. All these forceps should have very light springs to open their jaws. In case of strong spring the surgeon is unable to appreciate how firmly he or she is grasping the tissue. For holding skin, tough fascia or tendon, thumb forceps with a toothed tip

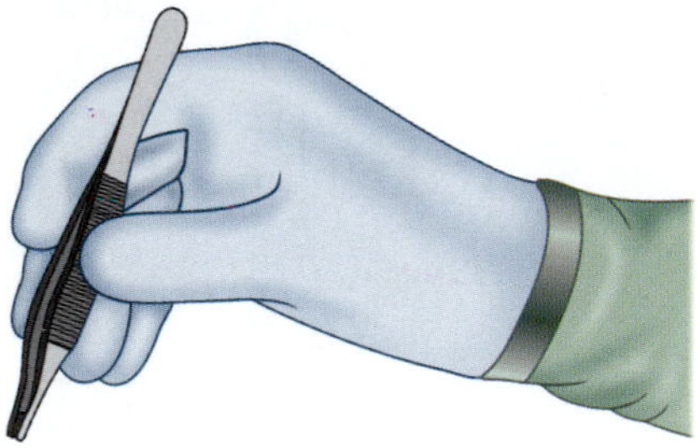

Figure 8.8: Method of holding thumb forceps

are used. For holding delicate structures, thumb forceps with smooth tips or serrated tips are used.

The main use of forceps is to retract, stabilise or grasp tissue. Forceps are held like a pen between the thumb and middle finger in the non dominant hand with index finger to stabilise the forceps (Fig. 8.8). Nontoothed thumb forceps with round tips may be used for dissection. The closed forceps tips are inserted into the desired plane and when the blades spring open, the tissue plane also opens.

Beside thumb forceps, there are other tissue holding forceps, e.g. Babcock forceps, Allis forceps and Lane's tissue forceps. Babcock forceps are non-traumatic and are used for holding the gut, ureter or bladder. Allis forceps have long blades with gaps between the blades. There are sharp teeth at the tip of the blades with grooves in between. When these forceps are locked, the tooth of one blade fits into the groove of the other blade and *vice versa*. These are used for holding tough structures such as skin, deep fascia or aponeurosis.

Lane's tissue forceps are heavy and traumatising, with curved fenestrated blades. At the tip, there is a heavy tooth in one blade with a groove in the other blade. In the closed position, the tooth fits into the groove. They may be used for grasping a fibrosed salivary gland during excision or the breast tissue during mastectomy. They may also be used to encircle the spermatic cord around its curved fenestrated blade during hernia repair, or as a replacement of a lost towel clip.

ARTERY FORCEPS (HAEMOSTATIC FORCEPS AND HAEMOSTATS)

These were devised by the celebrated French Surgeon, Ambroise Paré (1510–1590). His design was modified and improved by the introduction of a locking mechanism by Thomas Spencer Wells (1818–1897). Artery forceps are mainly used for holding bleeding vessels before they are occluded by a ligature or cauterised. They can also be used for dissection or for holding tough structures, such as fascia. They are pointed at one end, with rings at the ends of two shafts, linked with a hinge in the middle, and a ratchet to lock the blades.

Handling

Artery forceps and needle holders are held like surgical scissors (Figs 8.9 and 8.10). For locking the ratchet, handles are compressed. For unlocking, first lightly compress, and then separate the handles at a right angle to the hinge action. One should be able to lock and unlock them with either hand. For holding blood vessels, curved forceps are used with the concavity upwards and the tips extending beyond the vessel. For ligating blood vessels which have been held by artery forceps, the assistant holds the forceps tip facing upwards and visible, so that the surgeon can pass a ligature around the vessel. When the first

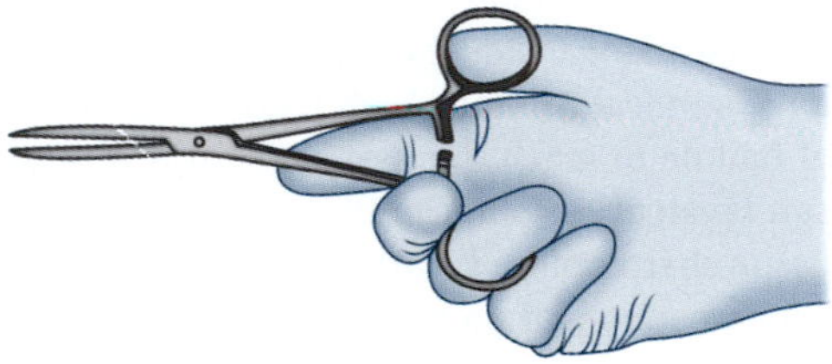

Figure 8.9: Method of holding artery forceps

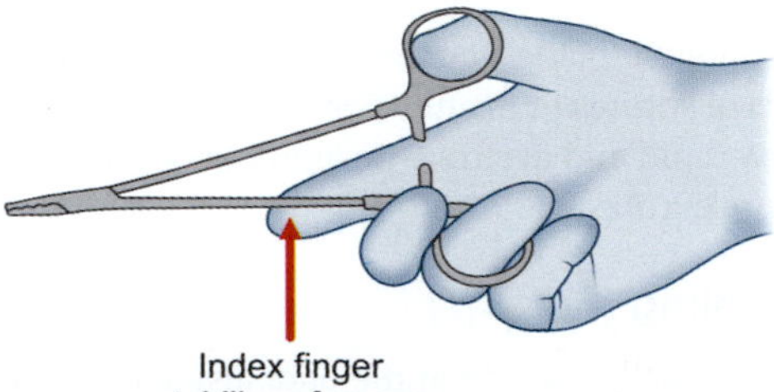

Figure 8.10: Method of opening an artery forceps

half of the knot is being tied, the assistant gently releases and removes the artery forceps only at the verbal request of the surgeon, and not before.

Artery forceps are available in different shapes and sizes. They can be either curved or straight. Small sized artery forceps with fine tips are also known as Mosquito forceps. Other types include Kelly's, Spencer Well's or Roberts. The Spencer Wells hemostatic forceps blades are usually half of the length of the shaft and have transverse serrations along the whole length of the blade with conical tips. In Kelly's clamps, the blades are short and transverse serrations are present along the whole length.

NEEDLE HOLDERS

These are used for holding and driving needles through the tissue. They may also be called needle drivers. A needle holder is held in the same way as the surgical scissors. It can be differentiated from artery forceps by smaller, short blunt blades, criss cross serrations and a groove in the centre of the blade for maintaining the orientation of the needle. A Mayo needle holder with a ratchet similar in design to that of artery forceps is commonly used.

Plastic surgeons may use a smaller needle holder without a locking device and with a scissor at the tip. This type of needle holder was devised by Sir Harold Gilles, the famous British plastic surgeon.

Handling

Needle holders grip needles with especially designed jaws (Fig. 8.11). Needles should be held at the junction of 1/3rd and 2/3rd of the way along the needle shaft from the suture material (Fig. 8.12). Pronation and supination (backhand and forehand) are used to drive the needle into tissue. During a pronation/supination movement, the needle holder rotates in its long axis and moves the needle in a curved plane through the tissue. A curved needle must be driven along its own curved shape through tissue, and will bend if gripped incorrectly, or driven in the wrong plane. Needles should be gripped at the tip of a needle holder, with a 90 to 105° angle with the shaft of the needle holder. The needlepoint should face the non-dominant hand and point upwards.

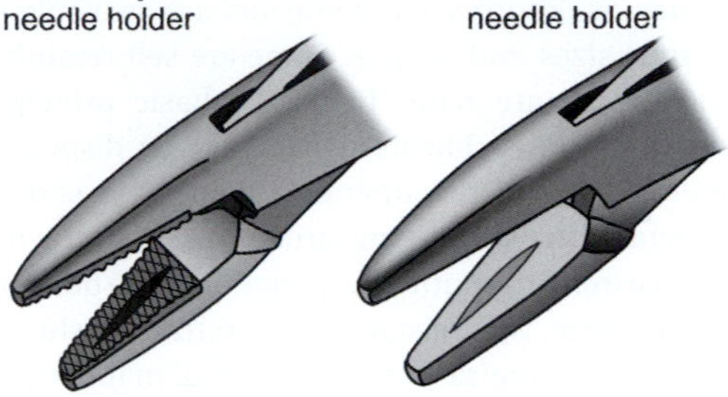

Figure 8.11: Serrated jaw and smooth jaw needle holder

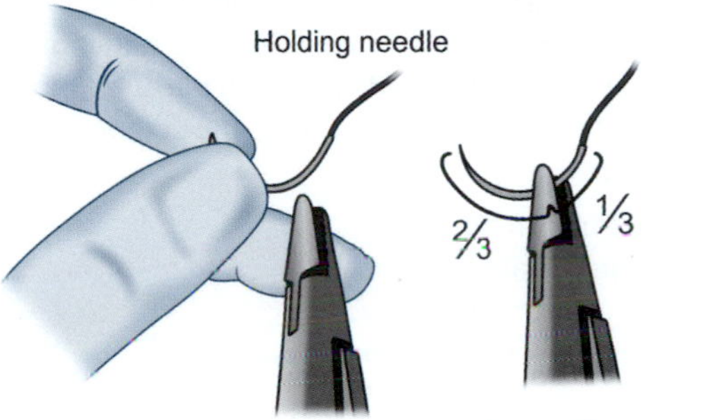

Figure 8.12: Holding needle with needle holder at the junction of 2/3rd and 1/3rd from it's tip

When suturing in a deep cavity such as the pelvis, it is a good practice to use long needle holders in order to avoid hands blocking vision of the needle and tissues. Whilst tying knots by hand, a needle holder with needle (mounted needle holder) may be kept on one side, in order to avoid a needle prick. Some surgeons palm the needle holder in the first interspace between thumb and second metacarpal, but this requires practice.

If it is essential to change the direction of a needle while stitching from right to left and *vice versa*, instead of taking out the needle from needle holder, turn the needle up side down inside the needle holder and then rotate the needle holder through 180° (Fig. 8.13).

RETRACTORS

Retractors are instruments used to pull tissue aside to expose a surgical field. They are especially useful when working in a close cavity such as the pelvis or on a deeply placed organ such as the kidney or oesophagus. Retractors are available in various sizes and shapes. Some are self-retaining and others are hand held. The basic principal of retraction is that tissues should be displaced laterally out of the operative field. One should safeguard the underlying structure to be retracted against injury by putting a sponge or gauze beneath the retractor. An assistant who is retracting should be allowed to relax between surgical manoeuvres in order to avoid fatigue and muscular cramps.

Retractors are used for traction, counter-traction or for both (Fig. 8.14). Traction is defined as pulling the tissue in one direction. Counter traction may be applied with another retractor or by hand, for example using a Deaver's retractor to retract the liver, and hand to retract the duodenum and bile duct in displaying the cystic duct structures.

Retractors can be:
- Superficial retractors
- Deep retractors
- Self-retaining retractors.

Superficial Retractors

1. *Langenbeck's retractor*: It has a long handle and small solid blade. It is commonly used for hernia surgery or in any superficial surgery to retract fascia or aponeurosis.
2. *Czerny retractor*: It has thick small blade on one side and biflanged hook on the other side in an opposite direction. It is used during abdominal closure while performing an appendectomy.

Deep Retractors

1. *Morris retractor*: It is used for abdominal wall retraction.
2. *Deaver's retractor*: It is used to retract liver, spleen and other abdominal organs. It is an atraumatic retractor and has a broad gently curved blade.
3. *Doyen's retractor*: It is used during pelvic operations.

Principals of Retraction

1. Retraction should be gentle.

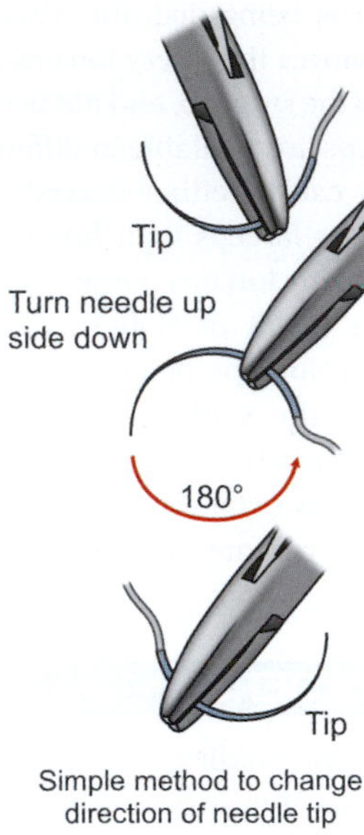

Figure 8.13: A method to change direction of needle tip

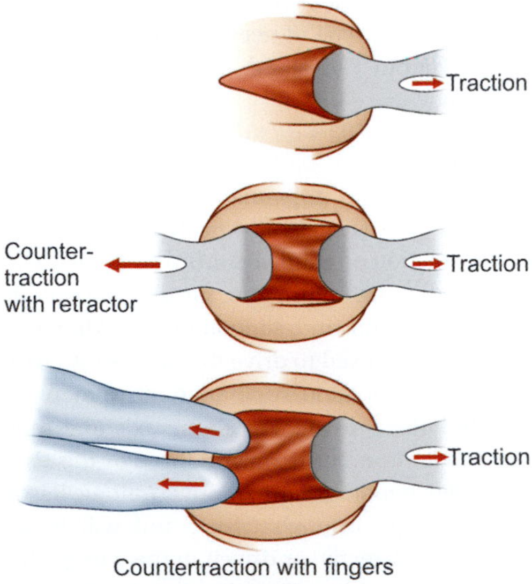

Figure 8.14: Traction by retractor and countertraction either by retractor or by fingers

2. Injury to underlying structures should be avoided during retraction.
3. During retraction of the abdominal wall, force should be directed laterally and upwards.

CLAMPS

Beside artery forceps which are used to permanently seal vessels, there are many other clamps with different uses in surgery.

Vascular clamps—for example, Bulldog clamp, Pott's arterial clamp and Satinsky clamps. These are designed to occlude vessels temporarily without damaging them.

Intestinal clamps—These can be crushing or noncrushing. Crushing clamps are used during intestinal resection to control bleeding and leakage from the divided bowel and to create a clean edge for anastomosis. Noncrushing intestinal clamps may be used to hold a viscus, and to prevent intestinal spillage. They are not totally atraumatic, and should be applied and locked up to one ratchet only.

Key Points

1. Proper handling of instruments is of paramount importance for optimum surgical outcome.
2. Hold a scalpel like a pen if a small precise incision is planned.
3. If a long incision on skin is planned, a scalpel may be held like a table knife.
4. No 3 BP handle accommodates size 10 to 15 surgical blades.
5. No 4 BP handle accommodates size 18 to 24 surgical blades.
6. Scissors can be used for a variety of functions ranging from tissue dissection, raising skin flaps and separating tissue planes.
7. Hold scissors in a mid-pronated hand position with distal phalanx of thumb occupying the ring of the moving blade and distal phalanx of ring finger occupying the other ring. Ring should never go beyond the distal interphalangeal joint.
8. In a needle holder, the needle should be held at the junction of 2/3rd and 1/3rd from the tip of needle.
9. Never push a needle through the tissue, rather use a movement of supination and pronation of the hand to drive the needle through tissue along its own shape. knot is used the hands should cross after one throw to lock it and make it safe.

Drains in Surgery

9

Sudhir Kumar Jain, David L Stoker

DEFINITION

A drain is a device to prevent collection of fluid in a cavity or a closed space. This space may be anatomical or created by surgical dissection. The fluid may be pus, blood, serum, urine, biliary or pancreatic secretions, intestinal contents, lymph or air. A drain is employed for continuous drainage of fluid outside the body as fluid is better outside than inside the body.

The question whether to put a drain or not cannot be answered with confidence and some element of subjectivity always exists in putting drains. This is especially evident after cholecystectomy when some surgeons put drains in almost every case but the majority use them selectively. Authors believe that when ever in doubt one should put in a drain.

The following are indications for inserting drains—the list is not exhaustive, and some indications are relative:

Drainage of Pus

a. After incision and drainage of any large abscess
b. Drainage of empyema of thorax
c. Drainage of empyema of gallbladder
d. After drainage of infected pseudo-cyst of pancreas
e. After surgery for peritonitis (Controversial)
f. Image-guided pigtail catheters are inserted to drain any localised intra-abdominal collection or liver abscess.

When drains are employed for pus or in contaminated wounds they should be kept in place for 5–7 days, so that a sinus track can get established. The purpose should be to keep the track open as long as it is needed to prevent re-accumulation of infected fluids inside the tissues. Premature removal of a drain can result in a deep seated abscess.

Drainage of Blood

a. Hemothorax
b. After laparotomy for hemoperitoneum secondary to any etiology
c. Drainage of scrotum after operation for large hydrocele
d. Drainage of subcutaneous space following mastectomy, thyroid surgery or open surgery for large incisional hernias
e. After liver surgery
f. Radical excision of pelvic tumours
g. After cholecystectomy if there is spillage of bile or suboptimal haemostasis.

Drainage of Intestinal Contents/Bile

a. After anastomosis of intestinal viscus when there is increased risk of leak, e.g. in the malnourished or septic patient, or where blood supply is threatened. A drain may herald a leak, leading to early re-laparotomy, or institution of early conservative primary management.
b. After common bile duct injuries during cholecystectomy.
c. After restorative surgery for bile duct strictures.

Drainage of Pancreatic Juice

1. After pancreatic resection
2. After pancreatic trauma.

Drainage of Chyle

1. Chylothorax
2. Chylocele

Drainage of Urine

Surgery on the urinary tract where urinary tract has been opened and leak is likely to occur.

Drainage of Air

Intercostal tube drain is employed for pneumothorax. Common indications for inserting drain can be therapeutic or prophylactic.

Therapeutic Indications

- Tension pneumothorax
- Pericardial temponade
- Solid organ abscess
- Intraperitoneal abscess
- Skin or subcutaneous abscess
- Hemothorax
- Empyema
- Pseudocyst of pancreas if it is infected and there is no communication with pancreatic duct.

Prophylactic Indications

- Post-thoracic surgery—cardiopulmonary or esophageal.
- Post-abdominal surgery (including urological procedures) if leak is suspected or likely to occur.
- Post-orthopaedic joint surgery.
- Head and neck surgery.
- Any operation involving extensive skin dissection or creation of myocutaneous flaps, e.g. mastectomy, incisional hernia, latissimus dorsi flap.

TYPES OF DRAINS

Tube Drains (Fig. 9.1)

Tube drains permit the formation of a closed drainage system, as they can be connected to bags or reservoirs. There are multiple holes at the end of the drain. Suction can be applied at the end of tube drains.

Sheet Drains (Figs 9.2 and 9.3)

These consist of corrugated silicone material, or sheets forming parallel tubes (Yeates drain), in which fluid passes through and around the tubes. These drains are either exteriorised through a main wound or via a separate stab wound. They are fixed by either suture to the skin or passing a large safety

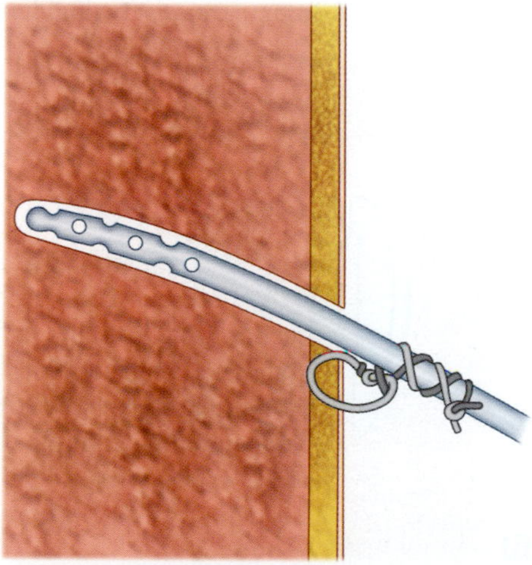

Figure 9.1: Tube drain with multiple side holes

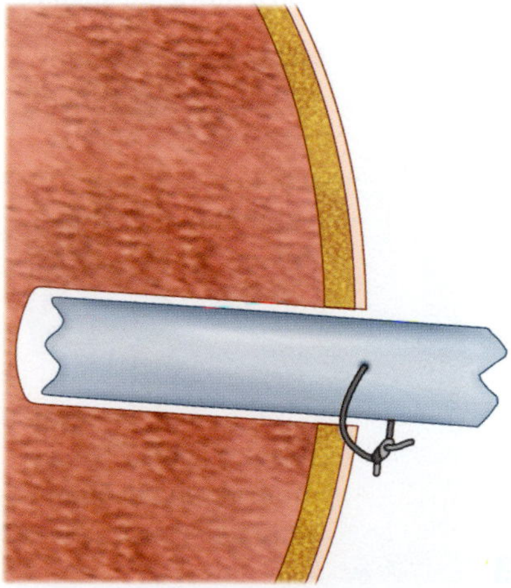

Figure 9.2: Corrugated sheet drain

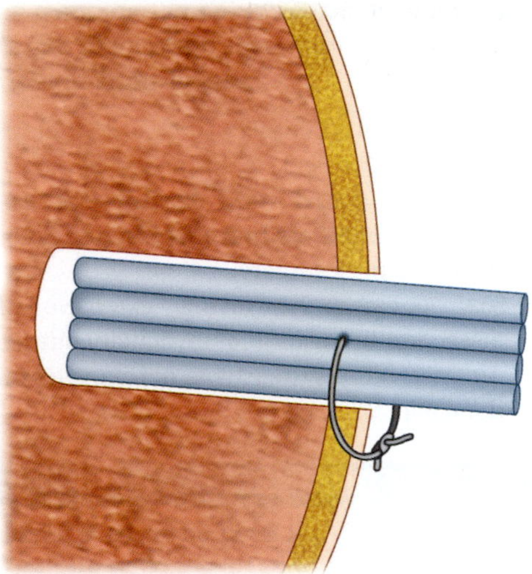

Figure 9.3: Yeates drain

pin through drain and skin. These drains are not used commonly in the present surgical era.

Gauze Packs and Ribbon Gauze Wicks (Figs 9.4A and B)

Gauze packs are sheets of sterile cotton gauze placed on a raw surface where discharge is expected to occur over a wide area, e.g. in an abscess cavity or after laying open of a fistulous tract. Gauze acts by capillary action, soaking up secretions. Packs may be soaked in saline with a lubricant such as liquid paraffin. Antiseptic agents such as betadine may also be used. Dry gauze packs are more effective but tend to adhere to raw areas and are difficult to remove. This may lead to pain and bleeding during removal. If a cavity is deep and discharge cannot be brought to the surface, it can be drained by a wick of folded gauze which is passed down. To be fully effective, it should be moist. Sometimes wicks can be passed through a thin walled latex tube, known as 'cigarette drain'. The latex tube prevents the wick becoming adherent to tissues (Fig. 9.5).

Drain can be made of:

1. *Latex rubber*: It is soft but excites a profound inflammatory reaction within 24 hours and renders them totally ineffective.
2. *PVC*: It is much less reactive and more efficient. It is firm and more unyielding but tends to harden with prolonged use especially when it comes in contact with bile.
3. *Silicon*: It is the best material for drains because it is least reactive, more pliable and does not get hardened with prolonged use.

TYPES OF DRAINAGE SYSTEMS

1. *Open drainage*: In this system Penrose drain, multitubular drain or corrugated drain is used. The drain is taken out through the main operative wound or via a separate stab wound stitched to the skin or secured by a safety pin.

   This is then covered by a surgical dressing pad. This type of drain increases the incidence

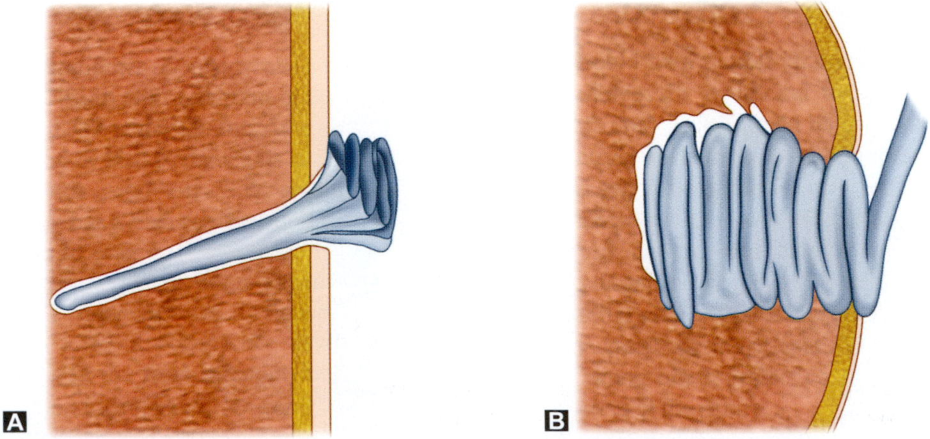

Figures 9.4A and B: Wound being packed by a folded gauze piece (A) or A ribbon pack (B) This is usually performed to drain a cavity

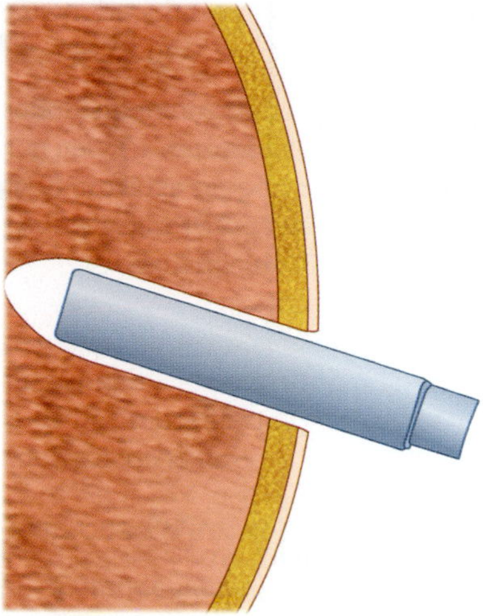

Figure 9.5: 'Cigarette' drain. This is formed by passing a folded gauze piece or a ribbon pack through a finger glove stalk or a thin walled rubber tube

of wound infection and disseminates infection to other patients in the surgical ward and is rarely used these days.

2. *Closed siphon drainage*: In this system a tube drain is connected to a drainage bag. The drainage bag has a one way valve at the entrance and a drainage tap at the opposite end. The tap allows daily emptying without disconnection.
3. *Closed suction drainage*: In this system firm polyethylene tubes are connected to portable suction devices. Some devices utilise low pressure vacuum (-100 to -150 mmHg), i.e. Romovac. Others utilise high pressure negative suction (-300 to 500 mmHg), i.e. Redivac. They are particularly used for drainage of dissected spaces, e.g. after incisional hernia repair. They should not be used inside the peritoneal cavity as they can cause injury to the gut due to negative suction.
4. *Sump suction drainage*: These drainage systems also employ negative suction but they have parallel air vents which prevent adjacent soft tissue from being sucked in to the lumen. They are made of either silicon or PVC. They are useful in management of small bowel fistula or pancreatic fistula.

Drains can be placed in the following anatomical spaces or planes:

1. Subcutaneous plane: Drains are inserted below flaps to take care of dead space. Common indications are after thyroid surgery, after mastectomy and ventral hernia repair. In these situations there is plenty of dead space and there are chances of blood collection in this space.
2. Intramuscular plane: After surgery for soft tissue sarcoma, e.g. compartmental excision.
3. After drainage of abscess: A drain is put in the residual cavity which prevents the premature closure of opening of abscess cavity and allows the abscess cavity to heal from below.
4. In the pleural cavity to drain blood, pus, air or infected fluid.
5. In the peritoneal cavity: After surgery for peritonitis, after major resection.
6. In the retroperitoneal space after renal surgery, after removal of retroperitoneal tumours.
7. In the retro pubic space to drain urine after bladder surgery, after open prostate removal.

Key Points

1. A drain is a device to prevent collection of undesired or unwanted fluid in a cavity or a closed space.
2. It can be used to drain pus, blood, intestinal contents, lymph or air.
3. Absolute indications for placing drains are tension pneumothorax, hemothorax, after pancreatic necrosectomy and in a localised collection of pus.
4. Drain may be harmful after appendicectomy.
5. A drain itself can cause complications by erosion into viscera.
6. Drains often reassure the surgeon rather than draining anything.
7. Whenever in doubt about hemostasis always put a drain.

Minimal Access Surgery

10

Raman Tanwar, Sudhir Kumar Jain, David L Stoker

DEFINITION

Minimal access surgery can be defined as the application of modern technology to minimise the trauma of surgical access, without compromising the exposure of the surgical site, or the safety of the patient.

INTRODUCTION

Wickman and Fitzpatrick in 1990 coined the term "minimally invasive surgery" in order to promote techniques with reduced operative trauma. Cuschieri in 1992 coined the term **m**inimal **a**ccess **s**urgery (MAS), which in many regards is more accurate and descriptive. The following techniques are included under the umbrella of MAS:

1. Laparoscopic surgery including conventional laparoscopy with use of multiple ports
2. Single incision laparoscopic surgery (SILS)
3. Hand assisted laparoscopic surgery (HALS)
4. Robotic assisted laparoscopic surgery
5. Video assisted thoracoscopy (VATS)
6. Natural orifice transendoluminal surgery (NOTES)
7. Endoluminal endoscopic surgery, e.g. surgery for early gastric carcinoma
8. Arthroscopic surgery
9. Minimal access thyroid surgery

   Minimal access surgery may not always be minimally invasive. Typical example for this statement is TEP repair of groin hernia which is a minimal access surgery in terms of incision but not minimally invasive as it requires extensive dissection in preperitoneal space.

In this chapter the basics of conventional laparoscopic surgery will be discussed.

The Advantages of Laparoscopic Surgery

In laparoscopy, retraction is provided by CO_2 pneumoperitoneum (8–12 mmHg), which is gently and evenly applied to the abdominal musculature and diaphragm, in contrast to the localised pressure of a mechanical retractor. Incisions are small at 5–12 mm in comparison to open surgery, and therefore less painful.

The incidence of hypothermia and evaporative fluid loss during laparoscopic surgery is much less because there is no exposure of the abdominal contents to the atmosphere. There is a lower incidence of postoperative intestinal adhesions after laparoscopy due to minimal handling of gut. Minimal handling of gut results in less serosal tears, less adhesions, and a reduced incidence of postoperative paralytic ileus. In the past there was a saying that "big surgeons make big incisions". A large incision, however, may be the cause of morbidity, increasing the likelihood of:

- *Postoperative pain (both acute and chronic)*
- Infection
- Bleeding
- Incisional hernia.

Any of the above may prevent early ambulation and recovery. Delay in mobility may lead to deep vein thrombosis, pulmonary embolism, or pulmonary consolidation.

Causes of Pain in Open Surgery include

1. Trauma of cutting muscles and other structures such as nerve, aponeurosis or fascia.
2. Mechanical retractors leading to localised bruising or ischemia to muscle or nerve caused by sustained pressure. A large incision is more painful than a small one.

All these are significantly less in laparoscopic surgery.

Following are Absolute Contraindications to Laparoscopic Surgery

1. Unwilling patient
2. Untrained surgeon
3. Untreated bleeding disorders
4. Patient in shock.

Relative Contraindications to Laparoscopic Surgery include

1. History of previous extensive abdominal surgery
2. Known intra-abdominal adhesions
3. Bowel obstruction
4. Pregnancy.

BASIC LAPAROSCOPIC SKILLS

Following skills should be learned by the novice laparoscopic Surgeon to take care of inherent limitations of laparoscopy.

Mechanical Limitations and Limited Degrees of Freedom of Instrument Movement

Currently available laparoscopic instruments offer only 4 degrees of freedom of movement, i.e. rotation, up/down, left/right angulations; in/out movement for straight long instruments and 6 degrees of movements for curved instruments. This limitation has been overcome by new instruments available for Robotic surgery which have 7 degrees of freedom with better perception of the surgical field. In contrast, in open surgery there is 360° of freedom of movement of instruments.

The limited degrees of freedom of movement make tissue handling with laparoscopic instruments more difficult. This is compounded with the fixed position of entry ports. Instrument changes during laparoscopic surgery are more laborious and distracting. Port sites should be planned very carefully and an experienced team will have no difficulty in changing instruments.

Less efficient instruments: A typical laparoscopic instrument transmits the force of a surgeon's hand from its handle to tip in ratio of only 3:1 in contrast to 1:3 ratios with a hemostat. The surgeon's hand therefore works about 6 times as hard to complete the same grasping task with the laparoscopic instrument. This is rarely a problem, and can be balanced by the fact that massively less retraction is required in awkward places.

Tactile feedback: There is a loss of direct tactile feedback because there is no direct contact of fingers with tissues. Indirect tactile feed back through instruments is markedly reduced due to the long length of instruments and because of friction between ports and instruments. This loss of indirect tactile feedback can lead to damage to tissue which has been grasped in an instrument, because the force which is being applied to grasped tissue is poorly appreciated by the surgeon's hand. This is true for a novice laparoscopic surgeon, and as the experience of the surgeon increases, this problem diminishes. Hand assisted minimal access surgery does not have this drawback.

Dark room: Operating room lights are turned off during laparoscopic surgery and the operating team works in relative darkness. Dark operating rooms during laparoscopic surgery increase the risk of collision hazards and using the wrong instruments. This can be overcome by providing a separate head light over the instrument trolley.

More clutter: The number of equipment, tubes and cables is greater during laparoscopic surgery in comparison to open surgery. This creates a hazard for traffic movement. Multiple tubes and cables may create a jungle of connections in the operating field if not well organised. This may decrease the efficiency of instrument handling, positioning and exchanges. In a well laid out modern theater there are neatly laid cables to the laparoscopic stack (Fig.10.1), and the only extra cables to the patient are the light cable and video lead.

***Tissue retrieval*:** Small port size limits the retrieval of solid or bulky organs, and sometimes a small separate incision needs to be made in order to remove organs, for example, colon. For solid organs a morcellator can be used, or tissue can be broken up into small pieces by finger fracture. These methods may risk wound contamination, or tumour cell implantation at port sites during retrieval. The risks are however low, and port site tumour recurrence should not occur if good surgical techniques are adhered to.

Skills to Overcome Visual Limitations

***Two-dimensional imaging*:** Standard monitors in current use are two dimensional imaging systems. The surgeon has to reconstruct three-dimensional pictures in his brain from the two-dimensional output. This includes intense perceptual and mental processing, which continues throughout a laparoscopic procedure. These days three-dimensional (3D) high definition monitors are available but they add to the cost.

***Limited view*:** There is a reduced field of vision and there is a decrease in the sensory input from the periphery of the field. There can be incidental tissue injury, when the instruments move outside the field of view. Movement of instruments within the abdomen must take place under direct vision to avoid accidental injury. This limitation is partly counterbalanced by the fact that the view is greatly magnified, and instruments can move anywhere in the abdominal cavity with ease.

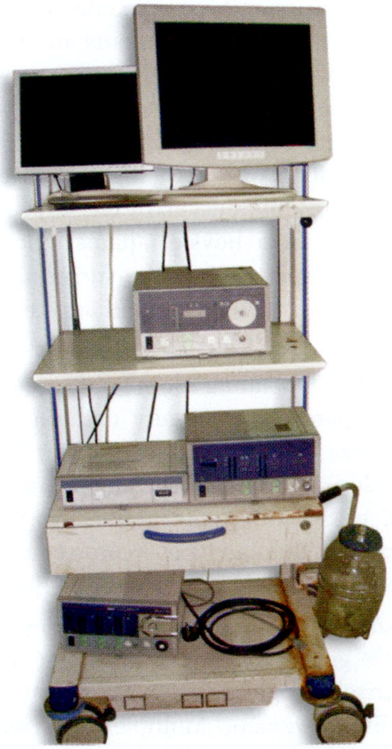

Figure 10.1: Showing laparoscopic stack containing video monitor, camera processing unit, insufflator, and light source

Decoupling of the Motor and Visual Spaces

The monitor should be placed in such a way that the visual axis formed between the surgeon's eyes and the monitor should be aligned with the hands and instruments. If they are not aligned it leads to poor task performance.

***Port placement* (*Fig. 10.2*):** Proper placement is extremely important for successful completion of a laparoscopic procedure. Manipulation angle,

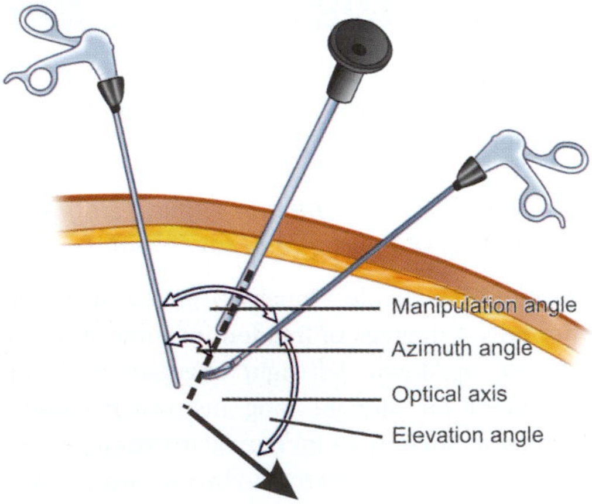

Figure 10.2: Physical axis and optical axis of a telescope

Azimuth angle and Elevation angles guide the site for optimal port placement.

Manipulation Angle

This is the angle between the active and assisting instrument. Manipulation angle should be between 45 and 75° with the ideal angle being 60° for an efficient performance of intracorporeal knotting.

Azimuth Angle

This is the angle between either of the instruments and the optical axis of the endoscope. Better work efficiency is obtained with equal Azimuth angles. Wide Azimuth angles should be avoided as far as possible.

Elevation Angle

This is the angle between the instrument and horizontal plane. Ideally the elevation angle should be equal to the manipulation angle. Ports should be placed in such a way that the ratio of intracorporeal and extracorporeal length of instrument should be 2:1. Ports for instruments and endoscope should be placed in such a way that instrument and endoscope are aligned in the same direction. One should not operate against the camera, because the surgeon will be working on a mirror image and manipulations become difficult in that situation.

Monitor Location

The monitor should ideally be placed in front of the surgeon and below eye level range (0 to 45°, 25° ideal) in order to produce a gaze down view. Gaze down viewing permits sensory signals and motor control to have a closed spatial location and bring visual signals in correspondence with instrument manipulations. The design of laparoscopic stacks is such that the monitors are usually at eye level.

Principles of Camera Operation

The camera operator's role is crucial in laparoscopic surgery because the camera is the eye of surgeon and surgeon will only see those things that are shown by the camera. The camera operator actively takes part in the surgery.

Golden Rules for Camera Operation

1. Keep the task in the centre of the field, which has best illumination and least image distortion, so that the surgeon sees the best quality image. Another reason for keeping in the centre is that if the surgeon works in the periphery of the field, instrument movement may take place outside the displayed image, and can accidentally damage adjacent structures.
2. If the surgeon wants better resolution of the target area for doing fine work, e.g. dissection or picking up a fallen clip, advance the telescope towards the target area, which will increase the resolution but decrease the size of visual field. During insertion of instruments or knot tying, a wider visual field is required and the laparoscope should be kept away from target area. When the surgeon becomes more experienced this may not be necessary.
3. Avoid jerky movements because they hinder precise surgery.
4. Keep the camera oriented at all times with a level horizon.
5. Before starting the procedure, do a white balancing of the camera and focus the camera on a gauze swab for reference.
6. During port insertion, keep the portion of the abdomen where the port will enter in the centre of the monitor field at all times to avoid injury to intra-abdominal organs.
7. During instrument insertion, the camera holder should guide the surgeon by showing a panoramic view for proper insertion of instruments. This becomes less important with a more experienced surgeon.

Selection of Laparoscope (Fig. 10.3)

Each endoscope has an optical axis and a physical axis. The optical axis is the axis passing through the centre of the visual field of the laparoscope. The physical axis is the axis passing through the centre of the endoscope. The endoscope can be 0°, 30° or 45° depending on the angle between optical axis

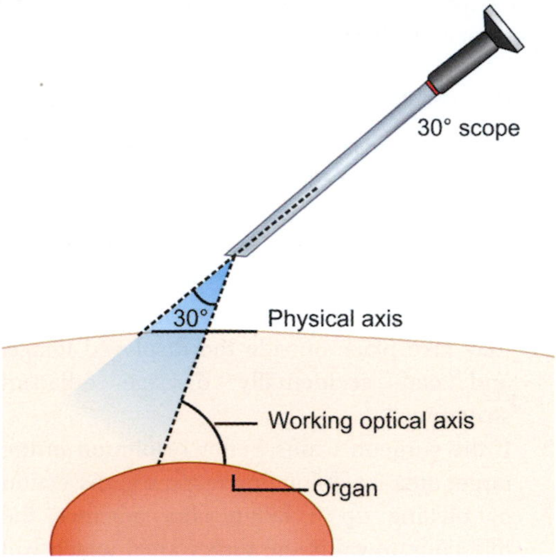

Figure 10.3: Various steps for inserting first port by open method

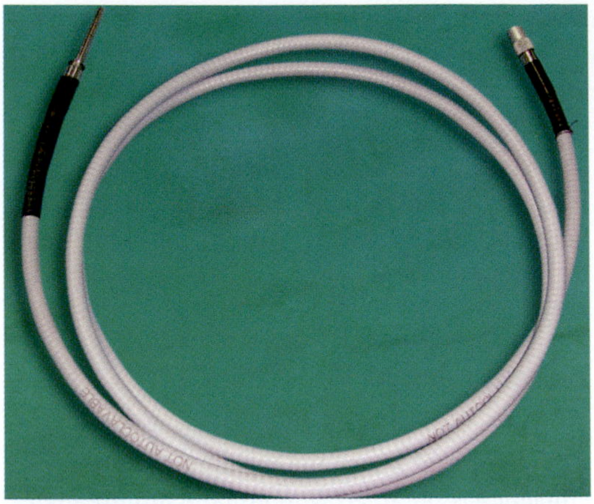

Figure 10.4: Showing fluid filled light cable

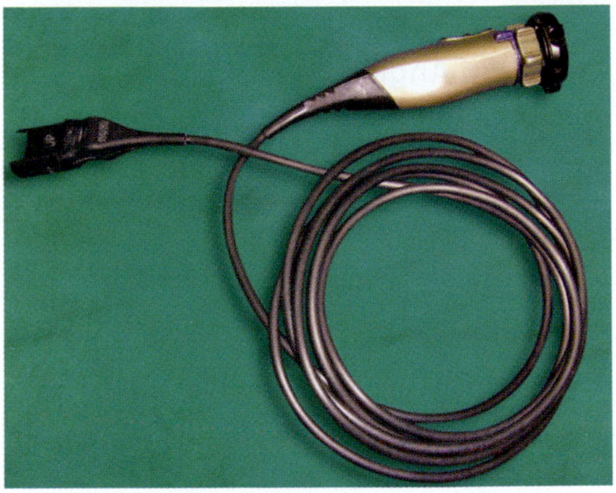

Figure 10.5: Showing camera head

and physical axis. The 30° laparoscope is useful in pelvic surgery and for difficult cholecystectomy. The 45° laparoscope is used for bariatric surgery and for surgery around the oesophageal hiatus. For common procedures a 0° laparoscope is sufficient. Camera angles can be changed during procedure by passing it through different ports thus improving the field of vision.

BASIC REQUIREMENTS FOR LAPAROSCOPIC SURGERY

Important basic equipment for laparoscopic surgery includes:

1. A rapid-flow insufflator
2. A light source
3. Video camera and camera cable (Figs 10.4 and 10.5)
4. A laparoscope
5. At least one monitor but two are desirable and add comfort to the assistant
6. Electrosurgical unit
7. Suction-irrigation machine
8. Laparoscopic instruments and ports.

The Rapid-Flow Insufflator

Carbon dioxide (CO_2) is used to create a pneumoperitoneum, creating a working space by distending the anterior, and lateral abdominal walls. CO_2 is preferred because:

It is an inert gas, and does not support combustion.

It is highly soluble, easily absorbed into the blood and easily excreted by the lungs.

It is readily available, inexpensive and nontoxic.

Automatic insufflators are used for insufflation of gas. These have a sensor, which can deliver a preset pressure of CO_2 and can control intra-abdominal pressure and rate of flow. Flow rate will increase if the intra-abdominal pressure falls below a preset level and flow rate automatically stops once the preset intra-abdominal pressure is reached. Modern automatic insufflators have bacteriological filters which can be incorporated along gas lines and can increase the temperature of the gas up to 37°, to prevent hypothermia during long laparoscopic procedures.

Light Sources

Light sources commonly in use are:

1. Xenon
2. Metal halide
3. Halogen.

Both xenon and metal halide give natural white light but the light of a xenon source is more natural. Halogen gives a yellow light, which is compensated by white balancing in the video camera system. All modern light sources have infrared filters. Commercially available xenon light sources can give an intensity varying from 150-300 lux. They have automatic intensity control which gives continuous optical illumination. Light from the source is carried to the laparoscope by a flexible light cable and down the laparoscope by a solid lens. Light cables are very delicate and should be handled with care.

Light cables can be:

1. Glass fiber light cable
2. Special fluid filled cable (Fig.10.4). Glass fiber light cables are more flexible but less efficient than fluid light cables because of fiber mismatch at the source or fiber breakage. Glass fiber light cables can be autoclaved but fluid filled cables should not be autoclaved.

Precautions to be Taken during Handling of Light Source and Cable

1. The light source should not be shone directly into the eye when unplugged from the laparoscope, as the very high intensity of light can cause retinal damage.
2. The ends of light cables can become very hot, with temperatures reaching up to 95°C, with the possibility of burns to anyone handling it. To prevent injury, the light source should initially be set on its lowest level (10-25%), and should be switched off when laparoscope is not in use. Light sources should have a fan to prevent the temperature rising too high and also to increase the life of the expensive bulbs.

Video Cameras

The cameras used in laparoscopy are miniature cameras based on a charged couple device (CCD). Chip camera systems have two components:

1. The camera head attached to the laparoscope.
2. The camera controller unit, which is located on an adjacent trolley which usually also holds the insufflator, and a monitor. The camera head consists of an objective lens and CCD chip. The lens focuses the image onto a CCD chip. The chip converts incoming photons into electronic charges and produces picture elements (pixels). This is possible because CCD chip is covered by a layer of light sensitive photoreceptors. The signal is then transmitted to the camera processing unit, where the image is generated for the monitor. There are two types of cameras, single chip versus three chip. In the single chip camera, only one chip processes all three primary colours. In three chip cameras, there is a separate chip for each primary color, i.e. red, green, and blue. This improves image definition.

PHYSIOLOGY OF PNEUMOPERITONEUM

Carbon Dioxide

CO_2 instilled into peritoneal cavity normally diffuses across the peritoneal surface into the venous circulation. After CO_2 is carried away by the venous system, it can be eliminated by the lungs or stored elsewhere in the body. The human body can store up to 120 litres of CO_2 and bone is the largest potential long term reservoir. Skeletal muscles and other potential visceral stores come into play if retention occurs for less than an hour. After storage, CO_2 is mainly eliminated by the lungs. Following a long laparoscopic procedure, it might take several hours for the accumulated CO_2 to be eliminated and for the body's acid base balance to be restored to normal. After laparoscopic surgery oxygen should be administered to assist in elimination of CO_2.

Carbon dioxide is used for insufflation because it is non toxic, colorless, noninflammable, non-toxic, readily soluble in blood and easily expelled from the body through the lungs.

Effects of CO_2

Direct local effects:
These effects include decreased cardiac output, pulmonary hypertension and systemic vasodilatation.

Centrally mediated effects:
Hypercarbia leads to widespread sympathetic stimulation resulting in tachycardia, vaso-constriction and increased central venous pressure, mean arterial pressure, pulmonary artery pressure and pulmonary vascular resistance. CO_2 causes transient hypercapnia and respiratory acidosis which is made worse with intra-abdominal pressure more than 12 mm of Hg and head down position. In healthy adults this can be compensated and also can be avoided by controlled hyperventilation and increased respiratory oxygen concentration.

Volume Effects of Pneumoperitoneum

1. Elevation of diaphragm, and anterolateral abdominal wall.
2. Decreased venous return due to increased pressure on the inferior vena cava.

Physiological Effects of Elevation of Diaphragm

1. Decreased functional residual capacity
2. Increased ventilation-perfusion mismatch
3. Increased intrapulmonary shunting
4. Increased alveolar-arterial gradient of oxygen partial pressure.

These effects are overcome by increasing the mechanical ventilation rate and concentration of inspired oxygen.

Physiological Effects of Decreased Venous Return

1. Initial increase in cardiac index followed by decrease in cardiac index (20–59%)
2. Cardiac axis of the heart shifts causing electrocardiographic alteration
3. 65% increase in systemic resistance
4. 90% increase in pulmonary vascular resistance.

These effects are overcome by an adequate volume load.

Metabolic Changes after Pneumoperitoneum

1. Four fold increase of renin and aldosterone.
2. Release of vasopressin, adrenaline and noradrenaline leading to sympathomimetic response.
3. Renal vasoconstriction leading to urinary sodium retention and temporary tubular renal dysfunction.
4. Hypothermia due to escape of water vapor along with gas leakage. Water vapor takes latent heat of vaporisation along with it causing heat loss. It is just like a wind blowing over the exposed abdominal contents. In prolonged procedure, core temperature can drop and hypothermia may result.

CREATING A SAFE PNEUMOPERITONEUM

There are two main methods of creating a safe pneumoperitoneum:
1. The closed method
2. The open method.

The Closed Method

A Verees needle is used to create a pneumoperitoneum. The Verees needle is a hollow needle with a spring loaded blunt centre core. The proximal end has a Luer lock which may be closed with a tap. The patency of the needle and spring loaded mechanism should be tested before using it.

The umbilicus is usually used for insertion of the Verees needle but in very obese patients or in patients with a history of previous abdominal surgery, the midclavicular point in the sub costal region of left hypochondrium can be used provided spleen enlargement has been ruled out. This point is also known as Palmer's point. In both areas, the needle should be held like a pen and directed towards the pelvic cavity rather than vertically downwards. Often, two "clicks" can be felt as the needle penetrates the abdominal wall, and the blunt trocar springs forward, firstly through muscle or linea Alba, then again through peritoneum. It is necessary to ascertain the safe position of the needle in the peritoneal cavity following insertion. The following tests are performed to make sure the Verees needle is in a safe position.

1. Attach a syringe to the Verees needle and aspirate. If intestinal contents or blood are aspirated, the needle should be withdrawn, as bowel or vascular injury may have occurred. In practice this happens rarely.
2. *The saline drop test*: A drop of saline put over the hub of the needle with the Luer lock opened, should be sucked inside the peritoneal cavity because of negative pressure. Saline should flow freely into the needle without difficulty.
3. Initial slow insufflation of CO_2 at a rate of one liter per minute should produce an initial intra-abdominal pressure of 5–7 mmHg. If the initial pressure reading is above 10 mmHg, the needle may be lying in the pre-peritoneal space, mesentery, or omentum. Once a safe pneumoperitoneum has been created, the first port insertion is usually via the umbilicus, directed towards the coccyx, preferably with a retractable blade to minimise the possibility of visceral damage.

In a variation of this technique, the laparoscope can be placed down the center of a different sort of port (Optiview, Visiport), with a transparent blunt tip, enabling the operator to see the tissues splitting, and the peritoneum opening *under vision*.

The Open Method (Fig. 10.6)

A vertical or horizontal 2 cm long infraumbilical incision is made. The incision is deepened down to the linea Alba.

The linear Alba is incised between stay sutures and peritoneum is exposed, and then incised for 1 cm *under vision*.

A finger is inserted inside peritoneal cavity to sweep away any adhesions, and a blunt tipped trocar is then inserted *under vision*. Stay sutures can be used to secure the port. Due to the size of the initial incision, gas leakage around the initial port can occur. A gas proof seal can be obtained by putting stitches around the port into skin over paraffin gauze, or a special port with occlusive balloons at the tip, known as a Hasson's cannula (Fig 10.7) can be used. The port has to be closed

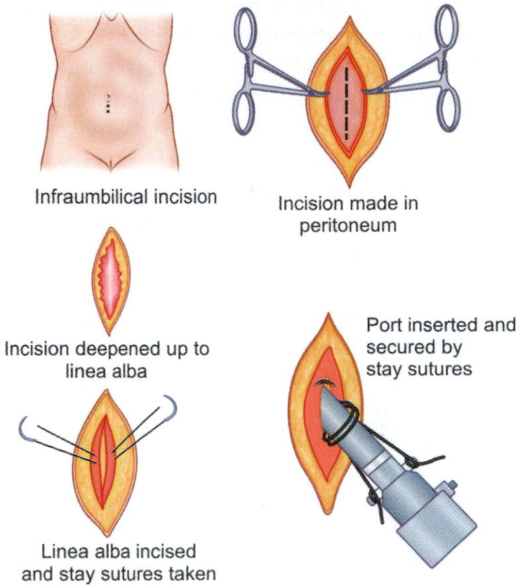

Incision made in peritoneum
Incision deepened up to linea alba
Port inserted and secured by stay sutures
Linea alba incised and stay sutures taken

Fig. 10.6: Various steps for inserting first port by open method

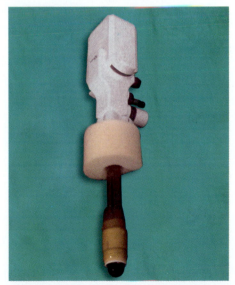

Figure 10.7: Showing self-retaining Hasson port used in open method of pneumoperitoneum

and repaired carefully at the end of the procedure, to prevent port site hernias developing.

The open method is now the most commonly used technique, as it has a lower incidence of bowel and vascular injury. It is not used universally, however, as the closed method is quicker, and produces a smaller scar. The serious vascular injury rate for the closed technique is in the range of 1:1000 insertions and practically nil by open technique. Incidence of bowel injury is much less with open technique in comparison to closed technique.

Summary of ergonomic physical recommendations for optimising the working conditions in laparoscopic surgery:

1. Foot pedal should be near the foot and at the same level.
2. Instrument handle should be at or slightly below elbow height.
3. Shoulders should be relaxed and arms should not be elevated.
4. There should be proper choice of instrument handle and grasp configuration for each task.

Key Points

1. Minimal access surgery is not always minimally invasive.
2. Proper selection of equipment and proper training is necessary before one embarks upon laparoscopic surgery.
3. Proper placement of ports is the key to success of laparoscopic surgery.
4. Safe creation of pneumoperitoneum is of paramount importance for starting of any laparoscopic procedure.
5. Open method for creation of pneumoperitoneum is safer than closed method with zero incidence of vascular injuries and a very low incidence of gut injuries.
6. There are mechanical and visual limitations of laparoscopic surgery which can be overcome by experience.
7. If intracorporeal suturing is planned, the manipulation angle between active instrument and assisting instrument should be between 45°–75°.

Haemostasis

11

Sudhir Kumar Jain, David L Stoker

The ability to control bleeding is an essential surgical skill which every surgeon must acquire. It is important during an episode of haemorrhage that the surgeon maintains his or her composure and controls bleeding without causing further damage to surrounding structures. One should always ask for a senior's help if one is not able to control the bleeding on his or her own. Galen (13 BC–200 AD) described several methods of controlling bleeding which are valid even today.

Drawbacks of excessive bleeding include:

1. Systemic complications like shock, clotting disorders, anaemia or impaired wound healing.
2. Retained blood in surgical field reduces visibility
3. Retained blood in wound provides culture media for bacteria which can lead to break down of clots and red cells leading to secondary bleeding.

TYPES OF BLEEDING

According to Source

1. Arterial bleeding is brisk, bright red, pulsatile and under high pressure.
2. Venous bleeding is dark red, continuous, low pressure, nonpulsatile, and difficult to control in comparison to arterial bleeding.
3. Capillary bleeding is a constant slow ooze from a raw area. It can usually be controlled by pressure.

According to Time of Bleeding

1. Primary haemorrhage occurs at the time of surgery or as a result of trauma. Bleeding may be excessive if there is an altered bleeding or clotting profile, e.g. liver disease, obstructive jaundice, malnutrition, haemophilia or if there is a disease involving arteries which prevents constriction of blood vessels, e.g. atherosclerosis.
2. Reactionary haemorrhage occurs within 24 hours of an operation. It usually occurs from small blood vessels from raw surfaces or from a minor capsular laceration of the staple line of anastomosis. Reactionary bleeding is usually caused by a rise in arterial or venous pressure leading to dislodgement of clots. This may be caused by pain, or excessive straining. Reactionary haemorrhage can occur after laparoscopic surgery, when small blood vessels compressed by increased intra-abdominal pressure start bleeding when the pneumoperitoneum is desufflated. Careful haemostasis is of paramount importance to avoid this problem.
3. Secondary haemorrhage usually occurs 7–10 days after surgery. It is usually due to an infection by organisms such as β-haemolytic Streptococci that cause dissolution of blood clots. Examples of secondary bleeding include bleeding from the tonsil bed after tonsillectomy, bleeding from an infected area after biliary surgery or bleeding from infected

vascular grafts. This type of haemorrhage may be secondary to autodigestion of blood clot following pancreatic surgery.

BLEEDING DURING SURGERY

During surgery some bleeding is inevitable. Blood loss tends to be greater during long or complex procedures such as liver resection, oesophageal resection, and major joint surgery. Every surgeon must acquire the skills necessary to firstly minimise blood loss, and secondly to control haemorrhage during surgery.

Prevention

1. In certain diseases such as obstructive jaundice, malnutrition, chronic liver disease and in haemophilia patients there is an increased propensity to bleed. In these situations, the bleeding and clotting profiles should be brought to normal. In obstructive jaundice and chronic liver disease intramuscular administration of 10 mg vitamin K often brings the prothrombin time to normal. In cases of emergency surgery, infusion of fresh frozen plasma often replenishes the deficient clotting factors.
2. If the patient is on oral anticoagulants, or heparin, these drugs should be stopped before surgery and the coagulation profile should be brought back to normal. Aspirin and other anti-platelet drugs should ideally be stopped at least 7-10 days before surgery.
3. Blood transfusion service protocols should be checked in order to decide if a blood sample is to be "Grouped and Saved", or if blood is to be cross matched. The availability of cross matched blood should be checked prior to surgery.
4. The technique of hypotensive anaesthesia may help minimise blood loss.
5. During head and neck surgery, raising the head end of the table 15-20° reduces venous congestion and blood loss.
6. While raising skin flaps during thyroid or breast surgery blood loss can be reduced by infiltration of normal saline or normal saline mixed with adrenaline (1:200,000). Fluid raises the tissue pressure, renders tissue transparent, and opens up the plane of dissection. Adrenaline produces local vasoconstriction and reduces the blood loss intraoperatively.
7. Revise the anatomy before starting any major surgery. This helps in identification of major blood vessels before they are injured.
8. If you are operating upon blood vessels or major organs, control of inflow vessels often helps in reducing bleeding. Noncrushing vascular clamps can be applied across the pedicle of an organ or the pedicle can be encircled with a tape prior to dissection.
9. If operating upon huge vascular tumors, e.g. renal cell carcinoma, preoperative embolisation of feeding vessels might reduce intraoperative bleeding, provided surgery is performed within 48–72 hours of embolisation. After 48 hours, there is development of new blood vessels which make surgery more difficult.
10. The tourniquet is a commonly used method for reducing blood loss when operating upon limbs. It is contraindicated in the presence of chronic ischaemia, impending gangrene, spreading cellulitis and in the presence of bony fractures. Before applying a tourniquet, the limb is emptied of blood by elevating it for 2-3 minutes. A pneumatic tourniquet is applied on the proximal part of the limb over orthopaedic wool. An Esmarch's bandage can be applied over the limb for more complete exsanguination, but it must be applied before applying the tourniquet. It is contraindicated in the presence of cellulitis. A tourniquet is applied around the upper arm or upper thigh over a thin layer of orthopedic wool and is inflated to 70-100 mmHg above systolic pressure (200 mmHg for arm and around 300 mmHg for the leg). It should be released after every 2 hours for at least 10 minutes before reapplying it.

CONTROL OF HAEMORRHAGE

1. Haemostasis by pressure:
   a. *Direct occlusion of hole in a vessel by finger tip* (Fig. 11.1): If pressure is applied by a

finger tip over a small cut on the vessel for 15–20 seconds a small clot will form over the divided end of the vessel and prevent further bleeding. The smooth surface of a moist gloved finger is less likely to dislodge the clot when finger is removed. If gauze is applied to the bleeding wound, clot is more likely to get dislodged as it can get adherent to the gauze.

b. *Pressure against underlying bone* (Fig. 11.2): If the incised skin wound happens to lie over bone, surgeons hand can be placed on the external surface of that wound edge

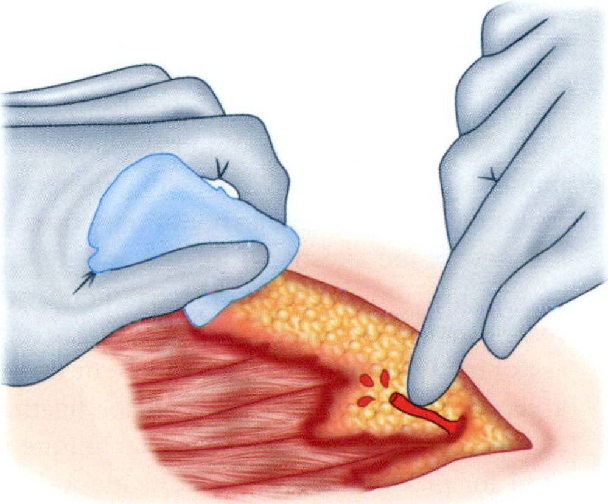

Figure 11.1: Showing use of finger pressure directly over vessel to stop bleeding

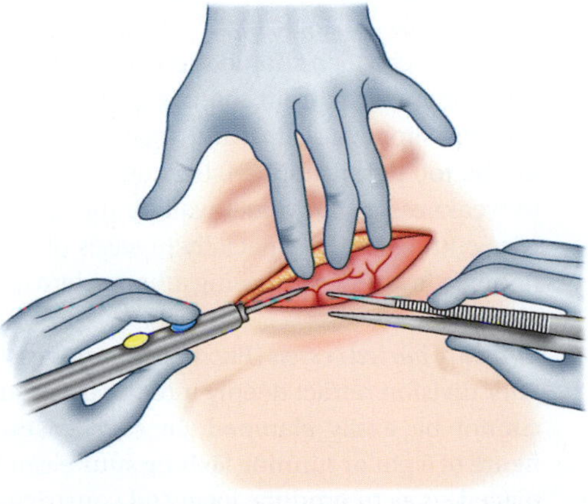

Figure 11.2: Control of bleeding by pressure against bone

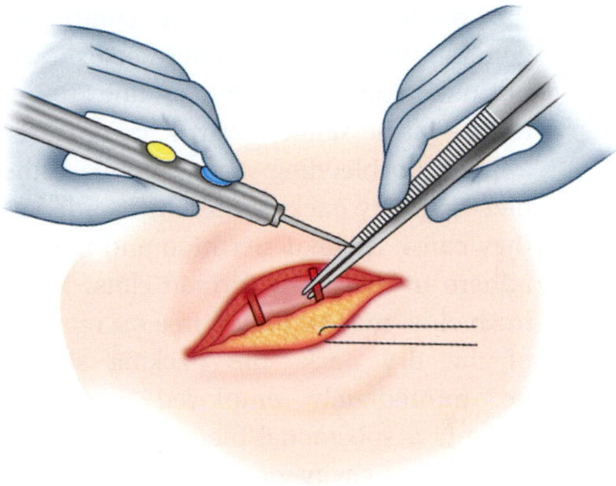

Figure 11.3: Showing control of bleeding by pressure of instrument

to compress the divided vessels against the firm underlying bone. Partial or serial release of that pressure will assist in identification of the open ends of any large vessel to be caught by artery forceps.

c. *Pressure with a knife or instrument tip* (Fig. 11.3): The tip of the knife can be used to immediately compress the open lumen of the vessel the moment it starts spurting during transaction by knife. The tip of the blade is quickly redirected to cover the cut vessel and to stop the bleeding until assistant grasps the bleeding point with forceps and cauterizes it or ligates it. The tip of the suction cannula can also be used in a similar manner by the surgical assistant to momentarily compress and arrest a bleeding point.

d. *Sponges* may be directly applied to a bleeding surface by the hand and fingers in order to arrest bleeding. If the bleeding occurs in a deep or narrow cavity where the hand cannot be put, a sponge mounted on a long handled instrument can reach up to the bleeding point to compress it until the surgical team is ready to clamp, ligate or cauterise it.

e. *Manual pressure* by packing or by a metal retractor over a pack is an invaluable method for control of bleeding. It is the method of choice for control of generalised oozing. The pack used should be moistened with cold saline rather than warm saline. Warm compresses applied on bleeding surface increase the bleeding. Dry packs should be avoided as they cause tissue desiccation and tend to adhere to the newly formed clots. These fresh clots may be pulled free on removal of the dry pack. The packing should be immediately employed whenever there is a substantial bleeding especially in a deep cavity or other inaccessible areas. Manual compression should be exerted over packs for 10–15 minutes observed strictly by the theatre clock. This manoeuvre provides immediate control, and the surgeon then has time to prepare himself for any necessary further action. Packing alone may be sufficient for certain clinical situations, e.g. extensive liver injuries. It also provides an opportunity for the anaesthetist to stabilise the patient. Manual pressure may occasionally be employed during laparoscopic surgery by using an atraumatic instrument or adjacent tissue over the bleeding area.

2. *Ligature and sutures* are the mainstay to control bleeding from large vessels (Figs 11.4 and 11.5). Clips and simple ligatures are commonly used methods of securing haemostasis. Both absorbable and non-absorbable material can be used to occlude divided vessels. Nonabsorbable materials are those which remain in the tissue for more than 60 days. These materials comprises of silk, cotton or metal clips, or vascular stapler. Absorbable material has some draw-backs of having less tensile strength and greater tissue reactivity. Absorbable materials also have poor handling qualities. However, in European countries where silk is no longer available, Polyglactin 710 is commonly used for ligation of blood vessels. In Asian countries particularly in India, surgeons prefer to use free silk ties for this purpose. Silk has best handling qualities and knot setting accuracy. However, because of its multiple strands and associated large surface area, it produces more fibrosis than monofilament sutures. Whilst tying the vessel, the hands of the surgeon should not obstruct the view of the assistant surgeon, and the tip of the instrument which has clamped the vessel should be visible all the time to the assistant. Two handed tie technique or tie on a clamp technique can be used for ligating clamped vessels. Tie on a clamp technique is used for tackling large vessels inside a deep cavity. Vessels of 2–5 mm in diameter can be occluded by clips or simple ligatures. Whilst applying a clip one should make sure that it surrounds the vessel completely. The clip should make an angle of 90° with the long axis of the vessel which should then be divided 3–4 millimeters away from the clip or ligature, to prevent slippage. Clips and ligatures should not be too tightly applied, because it can lead to weakness of the vessel wall by the cheese-wire cutting effect, especially in cases of rigid, nonelastic arteries following atherosclerosis in older patients.

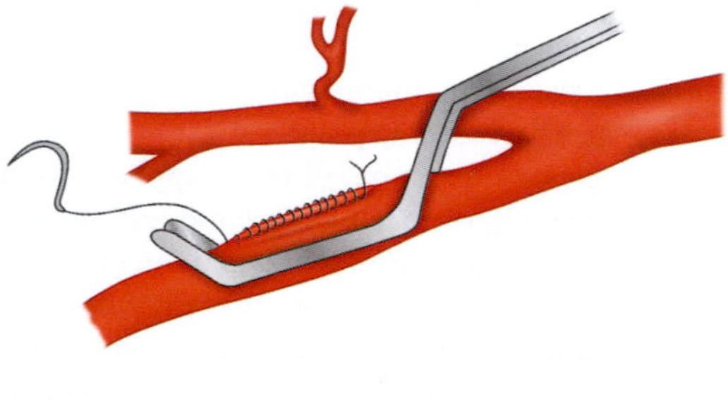

Figure 11.4: Showing closure of large rent in an artery by continuous suture

3. *Suture of buried vessels* (Fig. 11.6): Some vessels after division retract deeply into the tissue and cannot be easily clamped. In such cases, a figure of eight or running lashing suture can be placed so as to produce localised constriction of the cut surface along with the vessel.

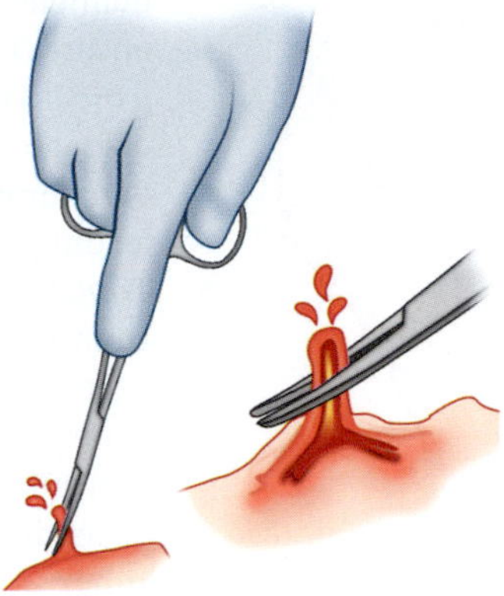

Figure 11.5A: Showing control of bleeding by artery forceps

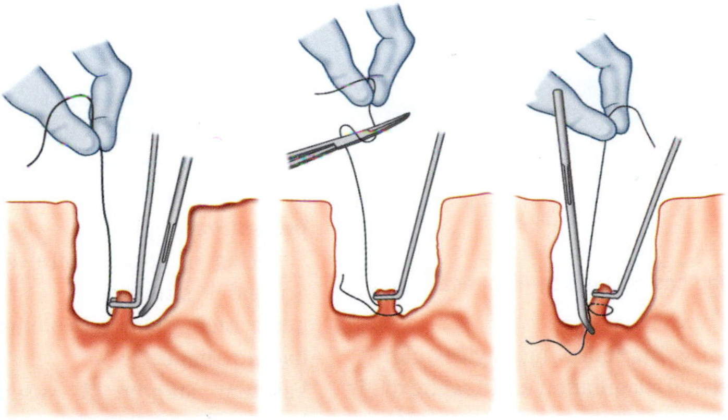

Figure 11.5B: Method of ligation of blood vessel held with a curved clamp with tip facing up

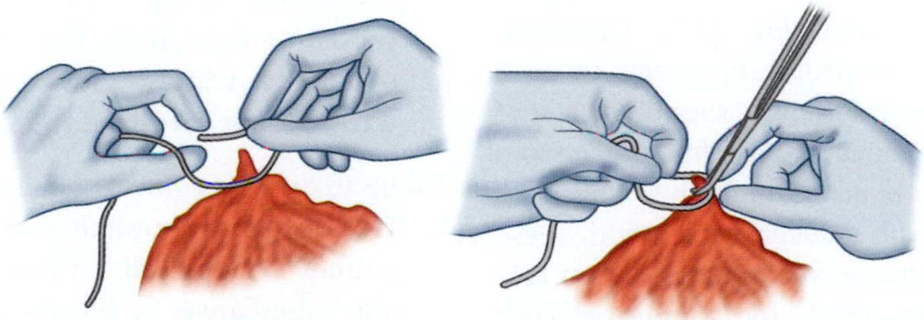

Figure 11.5C: Method of secure a bleeding vessel held with an artery forceps on the superficial surface

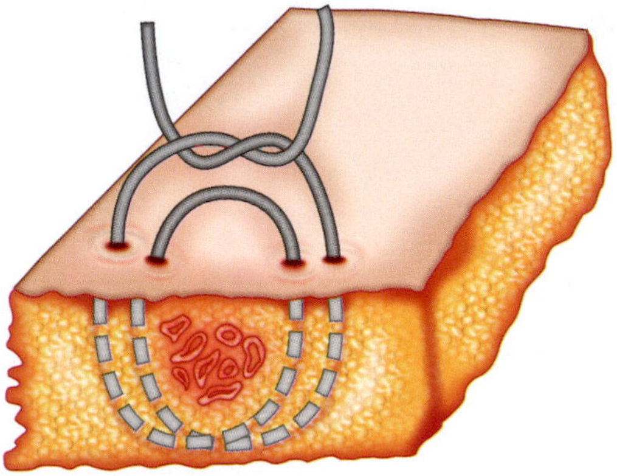

Figure 11.6: Showing figure of 8 sutures for control of deep seated bleeding vessel

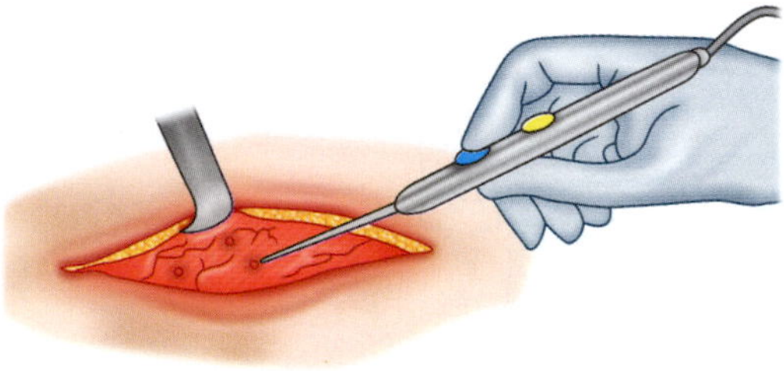

Figure 11.7: Showing haemostasis by electrocautery

4. *Energised systems*: The following devices can be used for thermal coagulation and sealing of blood vessels:
   a. Electrocoagulation
   b. Ultrasonic sealing
   c. Ligasure sealing
   d. Photocoagulation.

   Electrocoagulation is safe for sealing of vessels up to 2 mm (Fig. 11.7). Ultrasonic sealing is used for sealing of vessels up to 5 mm. Ultrasonic sealing uses sound waves not audible by the human ear, i.e. frequency more than 20,000 cycles per second. They cause less tissue heating with reduced penetration. These machines generate waves between 20–60 kHz frequencies produced by a piezoelectric transducer. They can cut, coagulate or separate tissue by high power density of around 100 W/sec and co-apt small vessels. The ligasure is used for sealing of vessels up to 7 mm in diameter. It provides a feedback loop that ensures complete sealing of the lumen before it breaks the flow of current. Photocoagulation uses an intense beam of light to produce denaturation and precipitation of proteins leading to coagulation.
5. *Transfixion and double ligature*: If an arterial stump continues to pulsate after simple ligature, this may indicate that the ligature is not safe and may slip due to the force of transmitted pulsation. Such a stump should be made safe by a transfixion stitch, in which either 2-0 or 3-0 Vicryl on a round bodied needle is passed through the wall of the stump, and tied on one side, then encircling the stump, and tied firmly on the other side with a surgeon's knot. Transfixation prevents the displacement of ligature. Transfixation and double ligature are generally needed for vessels over 5 mm in diameter, such as the femoral artery, splenic artery or renal artery. An experienced surgeon will often use a transfixion stitch on a large artery as a safety measure prior to division, during an elective procedure.
6. Suturing of stump: Suturing of a proximal arterial stump is still occasionally performed, using a Prolene stitch to prevent haemorrhage.
7. Vascular stapler: A vascular stapler can be used to provide a simple and safe way of dividing vascular pedicles during laparoscopic surgery. It may also be used in inaccessible areas during open surgery. The instrument fires three rows of vascular staples across the artery, and then cuts between the two staple lines. Vascular cartridges are supplied in white or grey colour. It is quick and effective, but very expensive.

Things to do after control of haemorrhage:
1. Do not close up immediately, but wait until the patient is stabilised, so that you can identify any other areas of bleeding which may not have manifested then due to hypotension.
2. One should wash out blood from body cavities with saline. Blood left inside a cavity can act as a nidus for bacterial proliferation and the

patient may also develop icterus in the post-operative period due to absorption of products of broken down haemoglobin.

3. Before closure, always make sure that you have not caused damage to other vital structures, e.g. damage to the common bile duct while controlling bleeding from a cystic artery.

Haemostasis with Drugs

Vasoconstrictors such as epinephrine and norepinephrine are quiet valuable in reducing blood loss. They may be injected in skin and subcutaneous tissue before making an incision. They should be injected at least 5–10 minutes before starting surgery as smooth muscle constriction in vessel wall requires 6 minutes to appear. A concentration of 1:200,000 epinephrine in saline is used and one can inject 40–50 ml of the solution in to an average adult weighing 70 kg. Caution should be exercised in using regional injections within or close to the pedicles of flaps. Advice of anaesthetist should be taken before injection of epinephrine. In long duration operations, the vasoconstrictor can be injected again after interval of 90 minutes.

Key Points

1. Every surgeon must be able to control haemorrhage during surgery.
2. In cases of unexpected bleeding keep yourself cool and composed.
3. Pack the bleeding area to buy time and organise yourself.
4. Inform the anaesthesiologist.
5. Do not hesitate to ask for a senior's help if you are not confident.
6. Wait for ten minutes before removing the pack.
7. After allowing sufficient time following packing, bleeding will often have reduced to a trickle to identify the bleeding point.
8. If packing does not help, proximal and distal control of a vessel may be needed.
9. If there is bleeding from a great vessel, suturing of a tear in the vessel may be required.

Biopsy Techniques

12

Sudhir Kumar Jain, David L Stoker

Biopsy is a process in which tissue is obtained for microscopic or other investigations. It is not analogous to fine needle aspiration, which obtains only cells. Fine needle aspiration is an alternative to biopsy but not a substitute, as there are many clinical situations in which there is no alternative to biopsy. Details of histological architecture and immunohistochemistry are only obtainable from biopsy specimens.

Indications for Biopsy

1. To confirm the diagnosis of malignancy, when there is strong clinical suspicion but repeated fine needle aspiration is not conclusive or negative.
2. In suspected cases of soft tissue sarcoma, lymphoma or follicular carcinoma of thyroid. In these cases fine needle aspiration cannot establish an exact diagnosis.
3. To differentiate between primary malignancy and metastasis.
4. In cases of breast malignancy where hormonal receptor status is required.
5. To differentiate between *in situ* carcinoma and invasive carcinoma.
6. Subtyping of malignancy for staging and prognostication.
7. In cases of testicular malignancy, if there are residual retroperitoneal masses post-radiotherapy or chemotherapy. Excision biopsy of residual masses is necessary to differentiate between residual malignancy and fibrosis.
8. Tissue is mandatory if any disease requires investigation with electron microscopy, enzyme histochemistry, and immunohistochemistry.

Enzyme Histochemistry is Required

1. For diagnosis of myopathy.
2. For diagnosis of malabsorption and alactasia.
3. For Hirschsprung's disease.

Immunohistochemistry is Needed

1. For sub typing of lymphoreticular tumours,
2. For identification of germ cell tumours (placental alkaline phosphatase),
3. Melanoma (by S-100, HMB45 and Vimetin),
4. Thyroid tumour (by thyroglobulin),
5. Vascular tumour (Endothelial marker, e.g. Factor VIII),
6. For identification of soft tissue tumours.

The Objective of a Tissue Biopsy is to Obtain a Tissue Sample

1. From a lesion which is representative of the pathology.
2. With preserved tissue architecture.
3. Should include a portion of normal tissue for comparison.

RULES OF TISSUE BIOPSY

1. In a large lesion, there can be areas of normal tissue in between lesions or lesion can be heterogeneous. To avoid sampling errors, one

should take multiple biopsies from different places.
2. In an ulcerated or fungating lesion, biopsy should not be taken from the centre, because this will most probably show necrotic tissue. Always take a biopsy from the periphery of the lesion, including normal tissue with it.
3. If it is surgically feasible and safe for the patient, always include the full thickness of the lesion in a biopsy to assess the depth of the lesion. This is especially important in staging of malignant melanoma.
4. Deeply situated masses may be surrounded by compressed normal surrounding tissue, forming a pseudocapsule. One should make sure that the biopsy traverses through this normal tissue in to the actual site of pathology before obtaining tissue. Failure to do so might result in a false-negative report.
5. Avoid handling biopsy tissue with crushing forceps or traumatic instruments, because this will lead to loss of tissue architecture, which is especially important in diagnosis of lymphoma.
6. Do not use laser or the cryoprobe whilst obtaining a biopsy, as they destroy tissue.
7. Do not use a morcellator for retrieving a solid organ after laparoscopic surgery, if you want a tissue diagnosis postoperatively.
8. Orientation of the resected specimen is important, if you need information on tumour free resected margins or staging. Orientation should be carried out in theatre by pinning out, or labelling with coloured sutures. This is of paramount importance in breast conservation surgery for cancer.

TYPES OF BIOPSY

1. Open biopsy
2. Percutaneous closed biopsy
3. Endoscopic biopsy
4. Laparoscopic biopsy

Open Biopsy

Open biopsy is usually performed for lesions in the skin and subcutaneous tissues. It is now unusual to open the abdomen or chest just for the sake of obtaining tissue.

Types of Open Biopsy

a. *Shave biopsy*: A scalpel or razor is used to shave off a thin layer of the lesion parallel to the skin.
b. *Punch biopsy*: A small cylindrical punch is screwed in to the lesion through full thickness and a cylinder of tissue is removed. Punch biopsy includes whole of epidermis/dermis and reaches up to subcutaneous fat. One to two stitches may be needed to close the wound.
c. *Incision biopsy*: Incision biopsy involves removal of a wedge of the lesion with adjacent normal tissue. Incision biopsy is used for large lesions prior to treatment.
d. *Excision biopsy*: In this, entire lesion is excised with a surrounding rim of normal tissue. This is used for small lesions, which can be excised completely.

Biopsy of Skin Lesions

Biopsy of skin lesions can be in the form of punch biopsy, shave biopsy or excision biopsy. Punch biopsy is indicated for flat or raised lesions (if melanoma is suspected). For pedunculated lesions, excision or shave biopsy is indicated. For a raised lesion, if melanoma is not suspected shave biopsy can suffice.

Indications for Biopsy in Oral Cavity Lesions

- Any lesion that persists for more than 2 weeks with no apparent aetiologic basis.
- Any inflammatory lesion that does not respond to local treatment after 10 to 14 days.
- Persistent hyperkeratotic changes in surface tissues.
- Any persistent tumescence, either visible or palpable beneath relatively normal tissue.

Characteristics of Oral Lesions that Raise the Suspicion of Malignancy

- Erythroplasia—The lesion which is totally red or has a speckled red appearance.

- Ulceration—If the lesion is ulcerated or presents as an ulcer.
- Duration—Any lesion which has persisted for more than two weeks.
- Growth rate—If lesion exhibits rapid growth
- Bleeding—If lesion bleeds on gentle manipulation or touch
- Induration—If lesion and surrounding tissue is firm to the touch
- Fixation—If lesion feels attached to adjacent structures.

Biopsy of Oral Lesion

a. Excision biopsy: Excision biopsy means removal of the whole of the lesion.
   Indications of excision biopsy are:
   - Should be employed with small lesions less than 1 cm.
   - The lesion on clinical exam appears benign.
   - If complete excision with a margin of normal tissue is possible without mutilation.

b. Incisional biopsy: An incision biopsy is a biopsy that samples only a particular portion or representative part of a lesion. If a lesion is large or has different characteristics in various locations more than one area may need to be sampled. The hazardous location of lesions is another indication for incisonal biopsy.

Percutaneous Closed Biopsy

1. Image guided
2. Blind

Image guided percutaneous biopsy is the method of choice, usually reserved for deep seated inaccessible lesions. Image guidance can be through ultrasonography or CT, and with the help of either, it is usually feasible to find a safe path or window through which the biopsy needle can pass into the region of interest.

Blind Biopsy

This can be used for superficial palpable lesions, kidney, liver and prostate. Various types of needles may be used.

1. Abraham's needle for pleural biopsy
2. Menghini needle for liver biopsy
3. Trucut needle
4. Automatic, spring loaded modification of trucut needle (Fig. 12.1).
5. High speed drill biopsy for bone only.

Endoscopic Biopsy (Fig. 12.2)

This can be used in association with both rigid and flexible endoscopy. Varieties of biopsy forceps are available. Since these biopsy forceps remove a very small amount of tissue, multiple biopsies at different points may need to be taken.

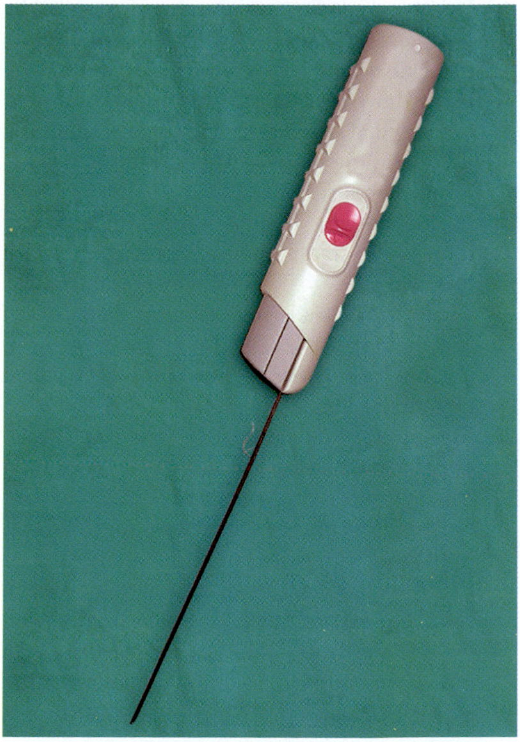

Figure 12.1: Trucut needle

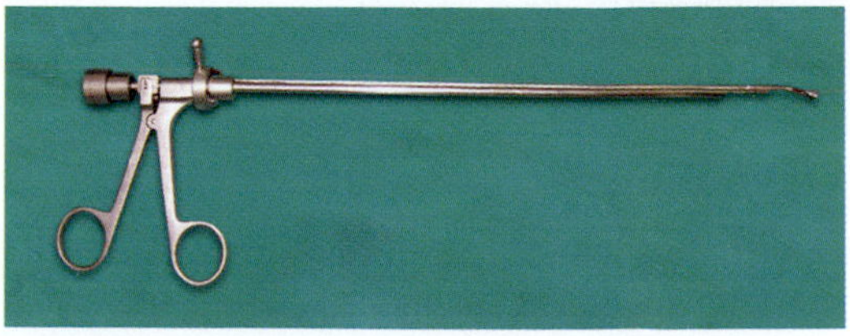

Figure 12.2: Cystoscopic biopsy forceps

Postbiopsy Procedure

1. A proper histology request form must be completed. Every specimen must be labelled correctly. The form must contain the patient's identification details, nature of specimen, clinical features, operative details and presumptive diagnosis. Patient details on the request form should match with the label on the specimen jar or container. Pathologists will also need to know if the patient had neoadjuvant chemotherapy for a full pathological staging report.
2. The specimen should be put in an appropriate fixative. Ten percent buffered formalin is suitable for most specimens.

Frozen Section

This is a special technique in which tissue is sent fresh to the pathology department, where it is frozen to -25°C using either liquid nitrogen or CO_2. After freezing, the tissue is immediately sectioned using a microtome in a special chamber known as a cryostat. Cut frozen sections are stained with haemotoxylin and eosin for immediate reporting. There has to be good coordination between the surgical and pathology teams when using this technique. Frozen sections are more difficult to interpret than ordinary paraffin sections and the services of an experienced pathologist are needed. It can be a highly accurate technique with false-negative rates of 0.5% and a false-positive rate of 0.1%.

Role of Frozen Section in Modern Day Clinical Practice

1. To establish the benign or malignant nature of a lesion during surgery, in order to decide on the extent of a resection. An example of this would be the management of solitary nodular goitre with fine needle aspiration report of follicular pathology. In this situation, the surgeon may perform a lobectomy and send it for frozen section. If the report is follicular carcinoma, he completes the procedure by doing a near total thyroidectomy. If the report is follicular adenoma, lobectomy itself is sufficient.
2. To ensure that resected margins are tumour free in malignancy. One of the examples is breast conservation surgery, in which the surgeon can revise the resected margins if not tumour free.
3. To establish that a biopsy contains sufficient material for diagnosis and is from a representative area in a difficult case.

Precautions to be Taken during Special Situations

Biopsy of an impalpable breast lesion detected by breast screening:

1. Preoperative X-ray localisation and insertion of localising needle under X-ray control, by the radiologist in a radiology suite is performed.
2. Suspected lesion with localising needle is removed.
3. Removed specimen along with needle is X-rayed and compared with preoperative mammogram film.
4. If image of removed specimen does not match with abnormality on mammogram, more tissue is removed.
5. Boundaries of removed specimen are marked with dye.
6. Removed specimen is sliced into serial 5 mm thickness sections on a special X-ray board and image again taken to determine which sections contain the exact lesion, which can then be further processed.

Lymph Node Biopsy

Which lymph node should be removed?

1. If there are involved lymph nodes in different anatomical areas, then choose an area which is more likely to be involved in the suspected pathology. For example in a suspected case of Hodgkin's lymphoma with involvement of cervical, axillary and inguinal lymph node, biopsy from an axillary lymph node will be preferred to that of a cervical or inguinal one.
2. If there are multiple lymph nodes in one anatomical group, then choose a lymph node which is least likely to be involved in nonspecific infection. Example is cervical lymphadenitis with involvement of submental,

submandibular and posterior cervical lymph nodes. In this clinical situation, biopsy from a posterior cervical group of lymph nodes is a more sensible choice because lymph nodes of submental and submandibular region are commonly involved in nonspecific infections of throat.

3. Choose a lymph node for biopsy which does not overlie or underlie an important structure. Excision biopsy is preferred over incision biopsy.
4. After biopsy the lymph node is bisected to inspect for gross pathology, i.e. caseous material, stony hard lymph node or lymph node containing pus. On bisection, imprints are taken on glass slides and stained. One half of the lymph node is sent in formalin for H and E staining. Remaining half is divided in to three parts. One piece is fixed in glutaraldehyde for electron microscopy. Another piece is snap frozen to –70°C for enzyme and immunohistochemistry. If infective pathology, e.g. tuberculosis is suspected, then remaining piece is kept in saline and stored at 4°C for microbiological examination.

Virtual Biopsy

Virtual biopsy refers to detection of tumour characteristics using a functional MRI or other imaging modalities to infer precise information regarding the size, extent and nature of the lesion. Using virtual biopsy the development of new vessels and the functional response to tumours can be studied. Brain lesions and colonic growths have been subjected to virtual biopsy with reliable results.

Key Points

1. In spite of advances in cytology techniques, biopsy techniques have a definite role.
2. Taking a biopsy is a basic surgical skill which every surgeon must acquire.
3. Tissue for biopsy must be taken from a representative area of pathology.
4. Excision biopsy is preferable to incision biopsy.
5. Avoid taking a biopsy from the centre of an ulcerating tumour.
6. Always include a portion of normal tissue while taking a biopsy from an ulcer.
7. Core needle biopsy is a good alternative to incision biopsy.
8. Always properly label biopsy specimens and give adequate details of clinical history and operative procedure to help the pathologist.
9. Send a biopsy specimen in the proper solution.
10. If planning for frozen sections inform the pathologist well in advance.

Dissection Techniques

13

Raman Tanwar, Sudhir Kumar Jain

DISSECTION

Dissection is an essential component for the successful completion of any surgical procedure. Quality of dissection is often judged as the hallmark of surgical competence. The technique of surgical dissection can be mastered by adopting sound surgical principals as well as by familiarity with surgical anatomy.

DEFINITION

Dissection is a Latin word derived from ('dis' meaning apart and 'secare' meaning to cut). It can be defined as "the exposure of a target organ or area by the process of separation of overlying tissue with haemostasis and preservation of surrounding essential or vital structures".

A good dissection requires not only a thorough knowledge of anatomy, but also a good understanding of the pathology of the relevant area.

Components of dissection:

1. Sensory component comprising of visual and tactile elements.
2. Access component involving tissue manipulation and instrument manoeuvre. The end point of good dissection is exposure of the target structure so that the desired procedure can be performed upon it.

Prerequisite of a Good Dissection

Application of the right amount of stretch on the tissues (without trauma) before starting to dissect. This entirely depends upon tactile feedback which the surgeon acquires during the initial years of training. Tension or stretching of tissues in the correct direction helps in identification of attachments and natural planes of separation.

Identification of Proper Tissue Planes

Economy of movement is very important. Each and every action the surgeon takes should be productive and should help in achieving the desired objective. Unproductive actions increase the chances of complications, and lead to fatigue. The surgeon should complete one step of the operation before proceeding to the next step.

MODES OF DISSECTION

Available modes of dissection are as follows:

1. Blunt dissection
2. Scissor dissection
3. Scalpel dissection
4. Ultrasonic dissection
5. Dissection by electrocautery
6. Hydrodissection by high velocity and high pressure water
7. Dissection by laser
8. Radiofrequency ablation

Blunt Dissection

Blunt dissection is suitable in places where there is a good amount of loose areolar tissue which can be separated by application of shear force. The safety of blunt dissection depends upon the sensitivity of tactile feedback to the surgeon's hands, which can differentiate between important structures, e.g. vessels or nerves and areolar tissue. Blunt dissection is especially useful in areas where anatomy is obscured.

Techniques of Blunt Dissection

1. Separation or splitting of overlying tissue. This is especially useful while dissecting along tubular structures such as vessels, nerves or ureter
2. Tearing or teasing of tissues
3. Wiping
4. Distraction
5. Peeling of over lying structures.

Methods of Blunt Dissection

1. Finger tip dissection: The tip of index finger allows living tissues to be opened without the need for excessive force. Finger tip dissection avoids heavy extertion by instruments. The use of heavy instruments can result in tearing of blood vessels, nerves and other structures with resultant heavy bleeding, loss of exposure and delayed healing. Surgeon's index finger can safely open avascular layers of collagen bundles which have formed at the site of previous scarring and can readily dissect many lightly adherent normal tissue planes. A tearing or shearing action can be performed by a finger along the line of separation. The tip of the finger can be used to peel off a structure, e.g. separation of gallbladder from its bed during cholecystectomy. Sometimes blunt dissection is performed by gauze wrapped on a finger, e.g. dissection of a hernial sac from the cord structures during inguinal hernia repair or during axillary dissection in breast cancer. Finger fracture technique may be used for liver resection.
2. Sponge or gauze dissection: If the density and adherence of tissue is significantly more than the tip of moist gloved finger, then finger tip dissection will not open the desired tissue planes. In these situations if a moist gauze piece wrapped around surgeon's index finger is used, it will increase the coefficient of friction between the wound and finger tip and facilitate dissection. The movements of finger in this type of dissection comprises of firm push and rotation of finger tips starting on the deeper or more fixed tissue which is followed by supination of hands and wrist so that mobile tissues are stripped and lifted away from deeper structures. Peeling action can also be performed by a pledget of gauze (Kuttner pledget) held in a pair of forceps to peel off fibrous tissue. During cholecystectomy, dissection in Calot's triangle is very often performed using this method. Peanut dissection is more effective when the gauze pledget is folded in half before clamping (Fig. 13.1).
3. Closed scissor tips can be used as blunt dissector. This technique is commonly used during lysis of adhesions during laparotomy. Blunt tipped scissors are excellent for opening tissue planes if the tissues are too dense for finger or sponge dissection but not so dense for as to require a scalpel. The technique of spread, then look is used for scissor dissection in which blades of closed tip scissor are first inserted in tissue planes then the blades of scissors are spread to open tissue planes, followed by division of any residual tough fascia bands. Scissor dissection is both safe and rapid in the hands of experienced surgeon. Many small blood vessels get closed off and sealed the moment they are cut during scissor dissection due shearing action of blades.
4. Splitting action is often performed by the pointed end of scissors to separate muscle fibres without cutting them, e.g. splitting of internal oblique/transversus abdominis muscle during appendicectomy.

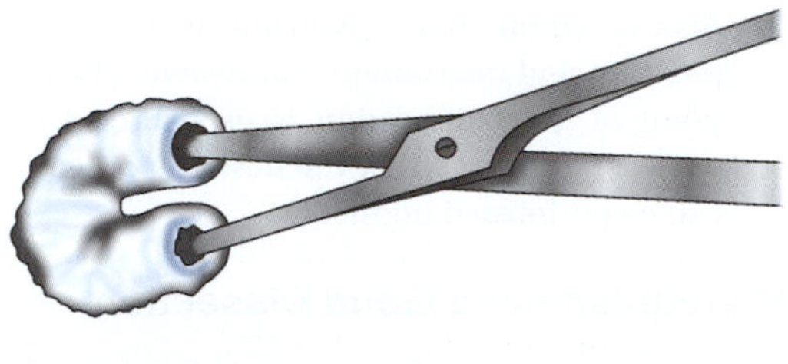

Figure 13.1: Kuttner pledget for dissection

5. Right angle forceps or Maryland dissector is commonly used for blunt dissection behind vascular bundles. It can, however, split, peel off or tear underlying structures, and therefore needs to be used with care.
6. Suction cannula is sometimes used as blunt dissection especially during laparoscopic surgery, often in conjunction with hydro-dissection.

Sharp Dissection

Sharp dissection involves division of tissues by cutting performed by scalpel or by scissors. Sharp dissection is a two handed procedure and needs application of the desired amount of tension by the nondominant hand with division and separation performed by the active hand. The technique of traction and counter-traction is often utilised whilst raising flaps during mastectomy or during thyroid surgery.

Knife dissection is used when tissues are heavily scarred or very dense. Sharp edge of the knife is used for this dissection. Knife dissection should be performed under exact visual monitoring otherwise it can result in damage to important structures. A blunt or dull knife should never be used because it makes cutting uncertain and excessive heavy pressure is needed to divide tissue. It will be difficult for surgeon to withdraw pressure immediately once desired depth of cutting has been reached resulting in damage to deeper tissues, e.g. to gut while opening abdomen. Scalpel dissection is performed by applying smooth horizontal strokes which deliver even pressure along the entire cutting edge. Small strokes with uneven pressure should be avoided as they result in more tissue damage, enhanced bleeding and increase operating time. Small strokes reflects uncertainty and indecisiveness in the mind of the operating surgeon. Special types of knives are also available for special situations. One such knife is Olive-tip or "button ended knife"—which can be inserted in a narrow space and used to make a lateral cut, e.g. lateral sphincterotomy in chronic anal fissure. Its rounded tip prevents any undesirable damage from the blade point thus making insertion of the knife in to a pocket safe and easy. Iridotomy knife used by eye surgeons is an example of such type of knife. Freer knife has a rounded edge at its tip and cutting is limited to that area only. It combines the features of a knife edge with that of sharp elevator and is particularly helpful in tangential undercutting to raise skin or mucous membrane flaps. A double edged knife has a sharp tip and sharp edge on both sides. It can be inserted in a pocket and swept from side-to-side for rapid undermining. These special knives are rarely used now and are of academic and historical interest only.

Diathermy Dissection

There are two types of handheld diathermy used commonly for dissection.

1. Handheld disposable diathermy probe with cutting and coagulation buttons. This is frequently used instead of scissors to divide tissues, and coagulate small vessels simultaneously. It facilitates a bloodless field, and has to be used carefully in the abdomen to avoid diathermy injury to bowel.
2. Monopolar and bipolar scissors. These are of the McIndoe variety, and come in various lengths for superficial or deep dissection. They combine the dissecting properties of McIndoe scissors with the properties of the handheld diathermy probe. They are particularly useful during abdominal and neck dissections. The diathermy works from a foot pedal and can be used selectively for tissues such as peritoneum, and serosa. They are useful for dividing adhesions. The bipolar scissors are safer to use, as adjacent tissues cannot be damaged by diathermy. This is because the current passes between the two scissors blades. These scissors have a limited life as they cannot be sharpened, and have to be replaced after 20–30 uses.

Ultrasonic Dissection

Ultrasonic dissectors are of two types:

1. Low power system
2. High power system

The low power system (CUSA Selector) is used for liver surgery. These systems cleave water containing tissues by cavitation leaving organised structures with low water content intact.

The high power system, e.g. Autosonix, Harmonic scalpel. This cleaves loose areolar tissue and blood vessels up to 3 mm diameter by fractional heating, performs coagulating and cutting action at the same time. It uses mechanical energy in the range of 55,000 cycles/sec and acts by disruption of hydrogen bonds and formation of a coagulum. It produces less heat in comparison to electrocautery and causes less collateral damage and tissue necrosis. The tip of the instrument remains very hot for several seconds after use, and caution needs to be taken to avoid it touching and burning adjacent tissues such as bowel, or the surgeon's fingers. It also helps in simultaneous haemostasis by coapting large vessels.

High Velocity Water Jet Dissection

This type of dissection disrupts friable, soft tissue but leaves ducts and blood vessels intact. It also has the effect of washing away adherent clot, which makes identification of anatomy much easier, e.g in dissection of Calot's triangle.

Laser Dissection

A variety of lasers may be used in surgery for dissection. Laser light is used to heat a probe to *white heat*, for example, a sapphire crystal. This very intense heat is highly efficient at cutting dense fibrous tissue, and may help to produce an almost bloodless field. Lasers are very expensive, and need strict protocols to avoid the hazards of eye exposure in theatre. Training is required in their use in specialised situations. Types of laser used include CO_2 laser, Holmium laser, KTP laser, Nd:YAG laser. Holmium laser can be used for dissection in endourological procedures as in prostate removal for benign hyperplasia of prostate.

Key Points

1. Dissection is an essential component for successful completion of any surgical procedure.
2. Quality of dissection is the hallmark of surgical competence.
3. Good dissection requires application of the right amount of stretch, identification of tissue planes and economy of movement.
4. Dissection can be either sharp or blunt.
5. Various devices like diathermy, ultrasonic machine or laser can be used for dissection.
6. Blunt dissection is useful in places where there is plenty of areolar tissue and anatomy is obscured.
7. Blunt dissection can be performed by finger, pledget of gauze held in a forceps, closed scissor tips, or by Maryland dissector.
8. Sharp dissection involves division of tissues by cutting using scissors or scalpel.

Surgical Diathermy: Principles and Precautions

14

Sudhir Kumar Jain, David L Stoker

Cushing and Bovie during the early twentieth century introduced surgical diathermy. The fact that whenever an electrical current passes through our body it induces intense neuromuscular stimulation and alteration of cardiac rhythm was described by Michel Faraday. With the increase in the frequency of alternating current, neuromuscular stimulation decreases and disappears at 500,000 Hz (50 kHz). Electrical diathermy units work on the principal of converting normal frequency alternating current (50 Hz) to high frequency alternating current (50 kHz). Modern day electrosurgical units can produce currents in the range of 200–300 kHz. Neuromuscular stimulation does not occur at such frequencies because current changes direction so rapidly that ionic exchange at cellular level does not occur, and muscle is not stimulated. High frequency alternating current, when concentrated on a small area, however, produces very high temperatures, capable of coagulating tissues.

Uses of Diathermy

1. For coagulation: Three types of coagulation modes can be used:
   a. Soft coagulation is the safest for both open and laparoscopic surgery. In this mode no electric arcs are generated between electrode and the tissue, as peak voltage is less than 200 V. In this mode there is shrinkage and desiccation of tissue without charring.
   b. Forced coagulation uses electric arcs to achieve deep coagulation. Peak voltages of more than 500 V are utilised to obtain this. This is useful in areas with high vascularity.
   c. Spray coagulation also known as fulguration in a noncontact mode which uses intensely modulated high frequency voltages (kV). A wider area of tissue is exposed to the current. Its main use is to control bleeding from an inaccessible vessel or to achieve haemostasis in a raw and bleeding area. The active electrode should not touch the patient's tissue during fulguration because in this mode the cell walls are destroyed through dehydration.

   For coagulation mode, current of *interrupted wave form of high voltage and low amplitude* is used. Cells walls contract using this mode due to protein denaturation and charring of cells.
2. For cutting, current of *continuous wave form of high amplitude and low voltage* is used. Heat production causes desiccation of cells due to water evaporation.
3. For blended mode, which can both cut and coagulate, amplitude and voltage of current are equal.

Modes of Diathermy

1. Monopolar (Fig. 14.1A)
2. Bipolar (Fig. 14.1B)

In monopolar diathermy, current passes from the generator via the active electrode (Fig. 14.2) through the patient and returns to the electrosurgical unit (Fig. 14.3) via a dispersive electrode (patient plate). In order to complete

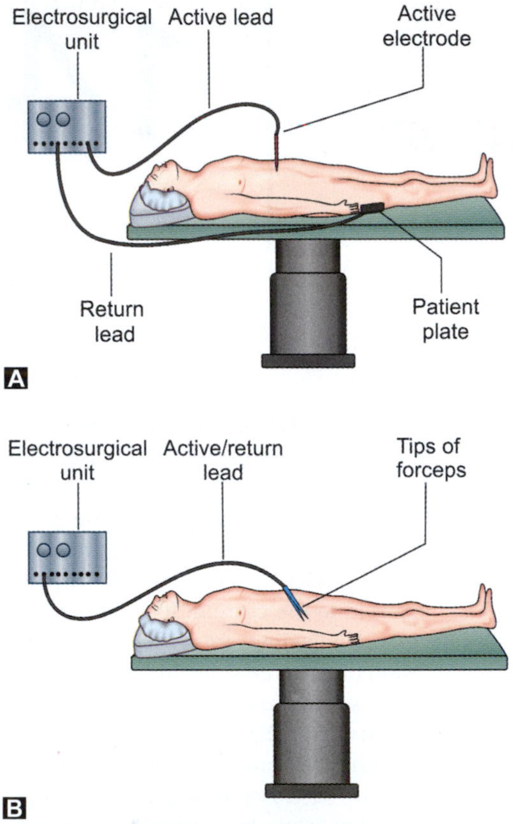

Figures 14.1A and B: Circuit of monopolar diathermy (A) and bipolar diathermy (B)

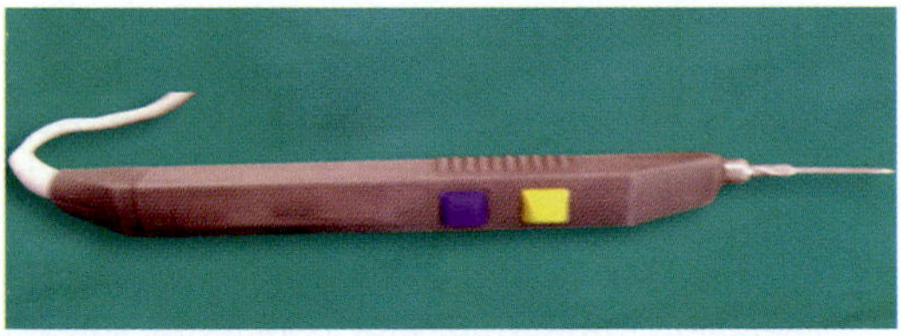

Figure 14.2: Showing hand operated electrocautery lead. Blue button for coagulation and yellow for cutting

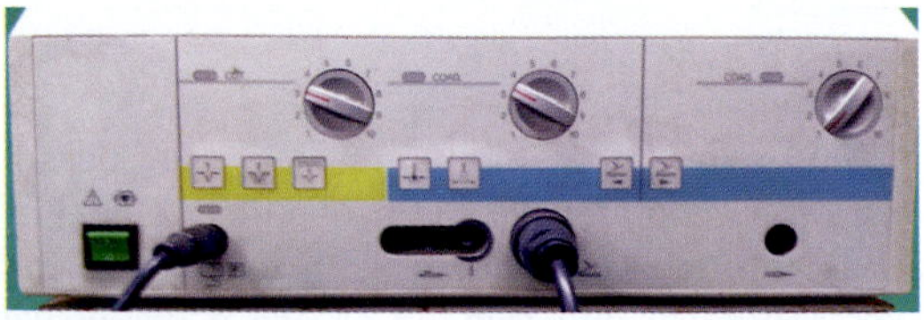

Figure 14.3: Showing electrocautery machine

the circuit and to return the current to the electrosurgical unit, a patient plate is always required. This should be in good contact with the patient's skin over at least 300 sq cm or more of area.

In bipolar mode, current passes from the generator to one prong or arm of bipolar forceps (or scissors), then through the patient tissue caught between the forceps and returns back to generator through the second prong or arm. The current does not therefore pass through the patient's body, as the circuit is completed through the bipolar forceps. This mode does not require a patient plate.

Uses of Bipolar Diathermy

1. When coagulation is required peripherally on an organ with a narrow pedicle, there is risk of channelling the current through the pedicle, leading to thrombosis of vessels, and a deleterious effect on the organ's blood supply. It is therefore, safer to use bipolar diathermy in this situation, e.g. circumcision.
2. When pinpoint or microcoagulation is required, e.g. neurosurgery, ophthalmic surgery, or plastic surgery.
3. When patient has a pacemaker *in situ*, in order to avoid problems that may be caused by a unipolar current passing through the heart.

Precautions when Using Diathermy

1. Equipment should be checked before use to ensure that it is in good working order. Regular check-up and maintenance of electrosurgery units should be performed to prevent injury to the patient and theatre personnel.
2. The diathermy plate or return electrode should be of an appropriate size (300 sq cm or more). The largest return electrode appropriate to the patient helps to ensure that electrical energy is not concentrated enough to generate significant heat and cause a burn.
3. The diathermy plate should be placed close to the operative site, and on the same side.

4. The diathermy plate should be placed over a well vascularised muscular area. Muscle is a better conductor of electricity, and good perfusion promotes electrical conductivity and dissipates heat.
5. If the skin at the site where the plate is to be placed is hairy, it should be shaved, as hair prevents complete plate contact with the patient skin.
6. The diathermy plate should not be placed over a bony prominence, scar tissue, skin over implanted metal prosthesis or areas distal to tourniquets. Bone is not a good conductor of electricity. Tissue perfusion may not be adequate in scar tissue. The plate can become over-heated if placed over an implanted metal prosthesis.
7. The diathermy plate should have a uniform and good body contact to permit the uniform flow of current.
8. There should not be any pooling of blood, body fluids or irrigation fluid near the diathermy plate, as this may lead to loss of contact due to moisture.
9. Patient's jewellery should be removed prior to transfer to the theatre as metal jewellery presents a potential risk of burn from directed current.
10. Contact of patient with grounded metal objects, e.g. IV stands, or anaesthesia machine should be avoided as they may become an alternate pathway for current leak to ground and can lead to accidental burns.
11. If there is a change in the position of the patient during surgery, the diathermy plate and wire should be re-inspected to make sure that there is no tension on the plate, which can result in reduced plate contact.
12. Alcohol based solutions should be avoided for preoperative skin preparation because they may ignite and increase the risk of a thermoelectrical burn.
13. The active diathermy electrode should be placed in an insulated quiver at all times when not in use.
14. The active electrode should have a secure tip. A loose tip may cause a spark. Eschar which builds up on the tip prevents the electrode from working safely, and regular cleaning during a surgical procedure may be necessary.
15. Electrosurgical smoke plume presents a potential biological and chemical hazard to both patients and staff. Smoke evacuation systems should be used for all procedures involving use of diathermy.
16. Monopolar units should not be operated in the vicinity of an electrocardiogram electrode (minimum distance of 15 cm) as they may lead to monitor malfunction.
17. Only the surgeon using the active electrode should activate the machine.
18. One should be cautious whilst using diathermy inside bowel. This is because intestinal gas contains the inflammable gases like hydrogen and methane which are potentially explosive.
19. Smoke plume generated from diathermy machine contains chemical by-products, e.g. toluene, benzene, hydrogen cyanide and formaldehyde which are potent carcinogens. Inhalation of these smoke plumes should be avoided by use of inline filters, use of special smoke evacuation systems or by use of improved surgical filtration masks.

Procedure for Starting a Monopolar Diathermy Machine

As the safety of monopolar diathermy depends upon proper placement of the patient plate, and only few diathermy machines have patient plate monitoring systems, one should adhere to the following procedures during start-up.

1. Place the patient plate on the patient at an appropriate place.
2. Connect the return lead to the patient plate.
3. Switch on diathermy machine, and plate continuity alarm will sound.
4. Connect return electrode to the diathermy machine, so that continuity alarm is silenced.

Hazards of Surgical Diathermy in Minimal Access Surgery (MAS)

Laparoscopic surgery has specific hazards in relation to electrocautery. These hazards arise due to the number of instruments and ports within the operative field.

The principal hazards are:

1. Insulation failure: This is the commonest cause of burns during MAS, and can be due to insulation failure, mechanical trauma, and repeated sterilisation of instruments or manufacturing flaws. Defects in the tip of the instrument within the view of the laparoscope can cause injury to a nontarget area, e.g. liver during laparoscopic cholecystectomy. Insulation defects in the shaft of an instrument can cause undetectable injury to any bowel it comes in contact with. Insulation failure at the handle of the instrument can burn the surgeon, or cause electric shock if the surgical glove is defective.
2. Capacitive coupling (Fig. 14.4): This is a phenomenon where an electrical current in the instrument induces a current in a nearby conductor in spite of intact insulation due to electromagnetic induction. This is because current flowing through an instrument induces an alternating magnetic field around it. There is increased incidence of capacitive coupling with higher voltages. It is of clinical significance in the following situations:
   a. Use of hybrid cannula, i.e. metal cannula within a plastic anchoring cannula.
   b. If an insulated electrode is passed through a metal port, there may be induction of current in the port, with up to 70% of current passing through insulated electrode.
   c. If an electrode is passed through the working channel of the laparoscope 70% of the current may be induced in the laparoscope.
3. Direct coupling: If an activated electrode touches another metal instrument there will be direct transfer of current from the activated electrode to the metal instrument. Tissues which are in contact with the metal instrument may be injured. Situations where direct coupling can occur are:
   a. Touching of an active electrode to the laparoscope.
   b. Touching of an active electrode to a metal clip or staple line.

Diathermy and Pacemakers

Diathermy currents can interfere with the working of pacemakers, which may be inhibited during diathermy activation, preventing cardiac pacing during cautery. A pacemaker may revert to a fixed rate of pacing during use of cautery and may require a magnet to reset it. If possible, the use of diathermy in a patient with a pacemaker should be avoided and other sources of energy such as the ultrasonic scalpel should be used.

If it is mandatory to use diathermy in such patients, the following precautions should be taken:

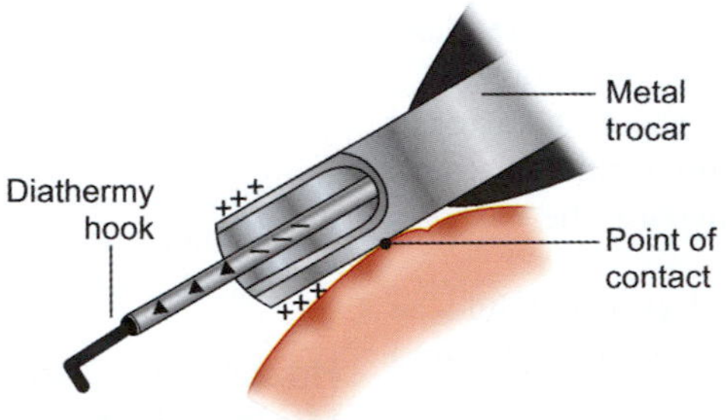

Figure 14.4: Mechanism of capacitative coupling by diathermy

1. Use bipolar mode, avoiding the use of monopolar diathermy.
2. If monopolar cautery is to be used, the patient plate should be sited in such a way that the current path does not pass through the heart or pacemaker.
3. Monitor heart beat throughout the operation.
4. A defibrillator should be available in case of dangerous arrhythmias.
5. Cardiologist should be asked to check pacemaker function prior to surgery.
6. Facilities for inserting a temporary pacemaker should be available.

Key Points

1. Diathermy uses high frequency alternating current (> 50 kHz) at which there is no neuromuscular stimulation.
2. Whenever current gets concentrated in a small area heat is generated.
3. One can use diathermy either for cutting or coagulation.
4. Cutting diathermy uses a low voltage, high frequency continuous wave form.
5. Coagulation uses high voltage, low frequency interrupted wave form.
6. Bipolar diathermy is safer than monopolar diathermy because the current does not pass through the patient's body.
7. Faulty position of patient's plate is the most common cause of diathermy burn.
8. Patient's plate must be well in contact with patient body over a well-vascularised muscular mass over a minimum area of at least 300 sq cm.
9. Avoid placing return electrode over scar, bony prominence, or distal to a tourniquet.
10. During laparoscopic surgery additional hazards of diathermy include direct coupling, insulation failure and capacitive coupling.
11. Do not use monopolar diathermy in a patient with a pacemaker.

Dressing and Wound Care

15

Gemma Conn, Sudhir Kumar Jain

Dressing of wounds is both an art and skill. A dressing can assist in accelerating the healing process if properly applied but also has potential of damaging the healing process. The surgeon must use proper materials and should acquire knowledge of how and when to use them. Dressings should be properly secured under tension, and should support the wound and give protection to it. The patient should not have an uneasy sensation and fear that dressings might come off unexpectedly during the postoperative period.

The art and skill of applying surgical dressings, these days are not taught to young surgeons. Hairy areas of skin should be shaved off before applying adhesive tapes. Tincture Benzoin if applied to surrounding skin before applying adhesive tapes increases the tape's adhesiveness and also protects the skin. Surgeons should remember that patients quite often view their dressings as a reflection of the skills and carefulness that proceeded before and during surgery, regardless of the fact that someone else has applied the dressing.

THE IDEAL DRESSING

The perfect dressing does not exist, however, if it did it would:

- Protect the wound from trauma
- Be impermeable to bacteria
- Allow oxygenation
- Retain moisture
- Be nonallergenic
- Not damage surrounding tissues.

Purpose of Dressings

1. *Wound protection*: Dressings serve the purpose of protecting the wound from external trauma or from patients own fingers. A simple absorbent gauze pad, well fixed with tape around the wound margin often suffices for this. In areas of open wounds gauze should be of fine mesh (30 μ) to avoid penetration of the gauze by ingrowing granulation tissue. Ingrowth of budding capillaries will cause pain on removal of dressings. Removal of coarse mesh dry gauze after several days of application will cause renewed bleeding because granulation tissue grows into the gauze and gets torn when the gauze is removed (Fig. 15.1).
2. *Promotion of wound drainage:* Use of moist or wet dressings will promote wound drainage by ensuring that fluids do not get trapped inside the wound. Moisture prevents the formation of scabs and crusts which usually occur if the wound is exposed to air. Liquids exudates are not thus blocked and will continue to escape into dressings in the postoperative period. This promotes normal mechanisms of wound healing by allowing drainage of harmful and necrotic material. Use of ointments or dressing material with ointment on wounds also reduces drying and crust formation. Ointments also prevent the dressing from

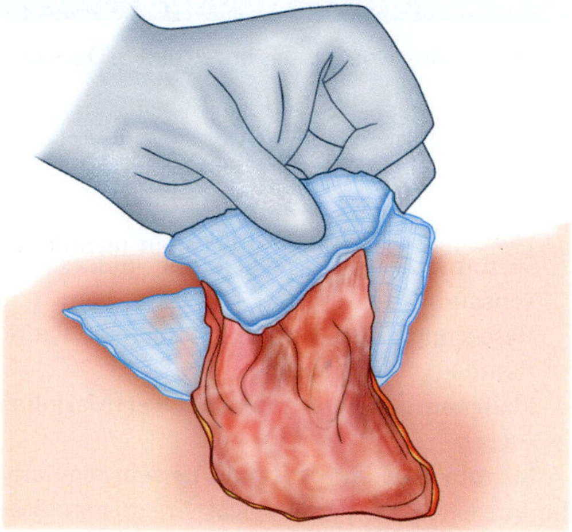

Figure 15.1: Granuation tissue grows into coarse mesh and can cause renewed bleeding on removal

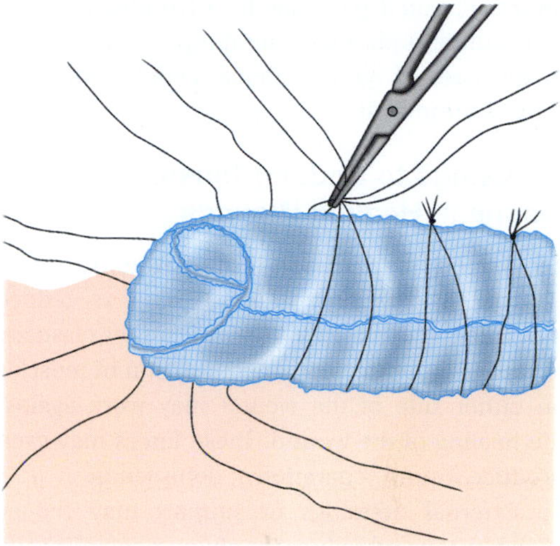

Figure 15.2: Tie on bolus dressing

adhering to the wound. Water soluble ointments should be preferred in comparison to oil based ointments as oil molecules can get trapped in wounds and act as foreign bodies leading to slowing of wound healing.

Dressings Intended to Kill Wound Bacteria

If the wound is expected to show a bacterial count of more than 10^3 per gram of tissue, a topical antibiotic ointment should be included in the dressing. Antibiotic ointment can be directly applied over the wound. Bacitracin is one such antibiotic which is well tolerated by living cells and seldom causes any tissue reaction. Neomycin or Furacin ointments can cause significant number of hypersensitivity reactions and should be used with caution.

Dressings to Splint the Wound

Many times dressings are applied to give rest to the body part during healing. Skin grafts require precise fixation and splinting during the first seven days after surgery so that graft can revacularise. Sudden displacement of the skin graft relative to the recipient bed during first few days will lead to disruption of tiny vascular anastomosis which are forming and the skin graft will fail to take up. Tie on bolus dressing (Fig. 15.2) is one of the best methods to dress skin grafts. This technique is of paramount importance at areas where involuntary movement is bound to occur, e.g. eye lids, lips, fingers, and neck.

Splinting of One Structure to Protect Another Part

A dressing may also be used to position one part of the body so as to use that part to protect or splint another. Example of this is the use of a dressing to fix the upper eyelid in a closed position to protect cornea from drying or injury in the postoperative period. To treat the fracture of the upper jaw, teeth in the non fractured lower jaw are wired ("dressed") against those on both sides of the fracture in the upper jaw.

Splinting of Painful Joints or Muscles

When muscles or joints are inflamed as a result of trauma, immobilisation by dressings may reduce discomfort and accelerate healing.

Dressings that Elevates a Body Part

Sometimes the function of the dressing is to simply elevate the part of the body above the heart to promote venous, capillary or lymphatic return. Elevated part may be a lymphedematous or cellulitic limb. Elevating the part may benefit in the case of lymphoedema, cellulitis or deep venous thrombosis.

Dressings to Reduce Tension on Tissue in Healing Wounds

Tension on the tissues in healing wounds can be reduced by splinting adjacent joints to reduce movements. It is a well-known fact that elasticity of the surrounding skin or contraction of muscles on either side of the wound may work against the healing of the wound. These forces may even produce wound separation or dehiscence.

External dressings or support may reduce such tension and reduce the chances retarding the wound healing. Following methods are used as anti-tension dressing:

- **Adhesive skin tapes (Fig. 15.3)**: Adhesive skin tapes are the most commonly used method for anti tension dressing. These tapes can be porous, or impermeable, rigid or elastic. Porous tapes have advantage that they permit drainage of serum and blood through pores. Tapes are used commonly to support a row of interrupted skin sutures, e.g. in thyroid surgery.
- **Elastic strip:** Elastic strip can expand to some extent if there is oedema of the tissues in wound after 2–3 days. Elastic tapes should not be applied in excessive tension as this can lead to blister formation.

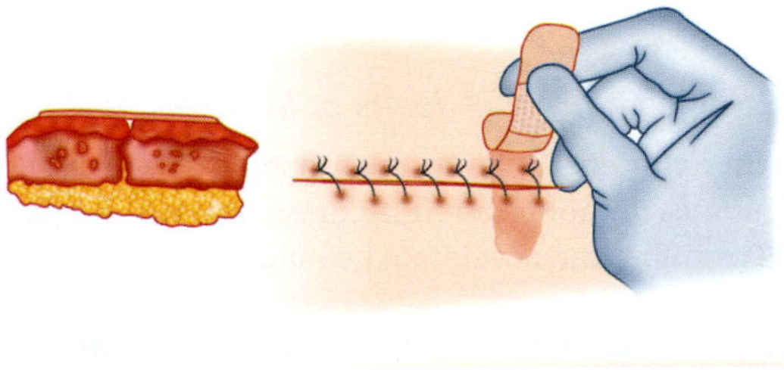

Figure 15.3: Use of adhesive tapes to reduce tension on wound

ASSESSMENT OF WOUNDS

When assessing wounds it is important to consider:
- Site
- Size
- Shape
- Depth
- Edges
- Surrounding tissues including pulses and sensation.
- Base-slough, eschar, necrotic tissue, granulation tissue
- Malignant change in a chronic ulcer (Marjolin's ulcer).

Microbiology swabs should be sent regularly. The presence of pathological organisms does not necessitate antibiotic treatment unless there is cellulitis or systemic sepsis. Regular dressing changes and debridement prevent bacterial counts from rising.

Necrotic Tissue

Necrotic tissue is devitalised or dead tissue. It is important to debride necrotic tissue to prevent infection, and enhance healing.

Slough

Slough is a mixture of dead cells, fibrin, serous exudates, white blood cells and bacteria. Sloughed wounds correspond to the proliferative stage of wound healing and it is important to encourage formation of granulation tissue. Large quantities of exudates can macerate surrounding tissues. If large volumes of exudate are present, then an absorbent dressing is required. If the wound is dry a dressing that retains moisture should be used.

Granulation Tissue

Granulation tissue is very vascular, resulting in a bright red colour. Dressings should be chosen according to the amount of exudates. Overgranulation prevents epithelialization and healing of the wound. It appears as prominent, friable pink tissue overgrowing the edge of the wound. It can be treated by application of a silver nitrate pencil.

Epithelialisation

Epithelial cells within the basal layer duplicate and migrate across a wound. A low adherence dressing should be used to avoid damage to these tissues. Dressing changes should be kept to a minimum, although it is important not to allow penetration of fluids through a dressing as this increases the risk of infection.

Exudates

Exudate contains leukocytes, enzymes, growth factors and cytokines, all of which are vital in wound healing. There is evidence to suggest that keeping a wound moist with exudate encourages healing.

Principles of Wound Care

When treating any wound it is necessary to consider:

- Nutrition status
- Pressure care
- Management of primary cause
- Drain sepsis/debride wound
- Treatment of cellulitis
- Cleaning the wound
- Promotion of healing
- Regular review by same group of individuals/team
- Documentation of progress.

Methods of Debridement

Autolytic

Autolytic debridement uses the body's ability to dissolve dead tissue. Dressings are used to enhance water retention in the wound, which traps enzymes, growth factors and other factors involved in healing.

Surgical

Debridement of necrotic tissues can be carried out in the ward during dressing changes. This should not be painful provided there is minimal inflammation of the surrounding tissues. More extensive debridement may require regional or general anaesthesia and must be performed in a theatre.

Biological

Larval therapy involves the application of sterile larvae to the wound, where they selectively digest necrotic tissue. Maggots do not damage healthy tissue.

Enzymatic

A pharmacologically developed version of collagenase has been developed that can aid digestion of necrotic tissue.

Mechanical

Mechanical debridement involves the application of saline soaked gauze to the wound. It is allowed to dry and is then removed the next day, removing with it the superficial layers of tissue.

TYPES OF DRESSING

Low Adherence

Low adherent dressings allow easy removal without damaging the wound or surrounding tissues. They allow exudate to seep through to secondary dressing. They are generally composed of perforated plastics, tulles or textiles, sometimes coated with a low adherent substance such as paraffin wax. Example of this type of dressing is Jelonet or Mepitel.

Semipermeable

These dressings are permeable to gas and water vapor, however, not to fluids or bacteria. These dressings are used in clean, dry or minimally exudating wounds. Opsite spray is a transparent film dressing spray which is permeable to gas and water vapor, but water-resistant. It is used on areas where a dressing is unlikely to adhere, e.g. flexible areas, fingers, or scalp. Examples are Tegaderm, Opsite and Mepore.

Foam

Foam dressings are composed of hydrophilic polyurethane foam. They are highly absorbent and can absorb heavy volumes of exudate preventing leakage onto surrounding skin. Allevyn, and Lyofoam are examples of this class.

Hydrocolloid

Hydrocolloids contain gel forming agents and form a gel on contact with exudate. They are used for absorbing mild to moderate amounts of exudate and promote autolysis. They are initially impermeable to exudate and bacteria. However, as the gelling process occurs, they become increasingly permeable to exudate. Aquacel, Tegasorb, and Granuflex are examples of this class.

Hydrogel

Hydrogels are water or glycerin based products, and therefore are gel like in consistency. They are used in cavities to promote autolysis of tissues in necrotic wounds. In dry wounds they are used to provide a moist environment, however, they can macerate surrounding normal tissue. These dressings are not used for exudative wounds as they exhibit poor absorption of exudate. They are nonadherent. Intrasite and Aquasorb belong to this class.

Antimicrobial

Antimicrobial dressings contain a topical antimicrobial agent which aims to reduce bacterial load. However, if a wound is overtly infected they will not convert it to a clean wound. Agents used include silver, iodine and metronidazole. They absorb small amounts of exudate. Aquacel Ag, Actisorb silver are examples of this category.

Capillary

Capillary dressings consist of a sandwich foam dressing that is highly absorbent and is therefore used for wounds with large amounts of exudate. These dressings damage dry wounds.

Alginate

Alginates are derived from alginic acid salts in brown seaweed. These dressings are used for heavily exudating wounds as they can absorb five times their weight in water. Alginates should not be used in dry wounds as they will stick, damaging tissue when removed. They are useful for dressing cavities. A secondary covering dressing is required.

Gauze

Used as a secondary dressing, often on top of low adherence/hydrocolloid dressings to absorb exudates. Also used on top of semipermeable dressings to provide pressure, reducing the risk of haematoma formation. They should not be applied directly to the wound as they will stick, damaging tissue when removed.

Waterproof

Waterproof dressings are permeable to gas but not to water vapor, fluids or bacteria. Therefore, they maintain a moist wound environment and so can lead to maceration. They are used over surgical wounds where there is a high risk of infection due to wound position (for example, over a laparotomy wound next to a stoma). Elastoplast is a waterproof dressing.

Vacuum Assisted Closure Device (VAC Pump)

The VAC pump applies low negative pressure to draw excess fluid from the wound, promote granulation tissue, aid wound contraction and reduce bacterial counts. A polyurethane ether foam dressing is cut to size and applied to the wound. The suction device is embedded within this and an adhesive, impermeable drape covers the wound and overlaps normal skin. The set up allows equal pressure to be applied across the whole wound. The evacuation tube is connected to an external canister in which the fluid is collected. These devices can be used on an outpatient basis but can also be effective in large wounds such as laparostomy.

Examples of Dressings in Various Common Clinical Scenarios

Necrotic Wound—Pressure Sore

The dead tissue in necrotic wounds loses moisture rapidly, and so often becomes hard and dry to touch. In order for healing to occur, this hard, dead, tissue must first be removed, either by surgical debridement, or by rehydrating the tissue thereby promoting autolysis. Typically a hydrogel, such as intrasite, is applied to the necrotic areas. A barrier cream is used on the edges to prevent maceration of the surrounding tissue. The area is then covered with a semipermeable dressing and re-inspected every 24 hours.

Sloughy Wound—Ulcer

The presence of a thick layer of slough predisposes to wound infection. Therefore, slough should be removed to promote healing, either by mechanical, biological or surgical debridement. Typically a hydrocolloid dressing is applied to promote autolysis and absorb exudates. For highly exudative wounds an alginate may be used. Gauze is then applied as a secondary dressing.

Granulation Tissue

For granulating wounds a low adherence dressing is used to prevent damage to the delicate tissue. A secondary dressing such as hydrocolloid/alginate is used to absorb exudates. Gauze is then applied to absorb any excess exudate.

Key Points

1. Dressing is both an art and skill.
2. Properly chosen dressing accerlerates healing.
3. Ideal dressing should protect wound from trauma and infection, be nonallergic, allow oxygenation of wound and should retain moisture.
4. Variety of dressings are available and one should choose according to the requirement of the wound.

Basics of Lasers in Surgery

16

Raman Tanwar, Sudhir Kumar Jain

LASER is an acronym that stands for **Light Amplification by Stimulated Emission of Radiation**. Laser is a light made up of monochromatic (one colour or wavelength), coherent, parallel photons moving in the same direction, which potentiates the amount of energy carried by it compared to white light. The wavelength and power output of the laser determines its application in terms of cutting, vapourizing or sealing tissues. These three properties of laser light, i.e. monochromaticity, directionality and coherence make them more hazardous than ordinary light as laser light can deposit a lot of energy within a small area. Aim of this chapter is to outline the basic fundamentals of laser and the precautions which should be observed during its use.

Common Components of all Lasers

Active Medium

The active media may be solids, liquid dyes or gases. Commonly used mediums are Ruby, Nd:YAG, CO_2 or Helium/Neon. Active medium contains atoms whose electrons may be excited to a metastable energy level by an energy source.

Excitation Mechanism

Excitation mechanisms pump energy into the active medium by optical, electrical or chemical methods.

High Reflectance Mirror

It is a mirror which reflects essentially 100% of the laser light.

Partially Transmissive Mirror

It is a mirror which reflects less than 100% of the laser light and transmits the remainder.

The earliest uses of laser in medical treatment dates back to 1961 when the first solid state (Nd:YAG) and gaseous state (based on helium and neon) lasers were developed. Consequently, the argon and the carbon dioxide lasers were developed within a span of 2 more years. Coumarin and Ruby lasers were some of the earlier lasers to be used in medicine, and have been replaced in the modern era by more efficient and flexible lasers with higher peak power.

Lasers exert their effect in various ways attributing to their unique properties. Of these the photothermal and photoablative effects are the most commonly exploited properties in the field of surgery. When used in delicate areas like the blood vessels or mucosa the laser can cause ablation of tissue which can be precisely controlled. This is often referred to as the photoablative effect. Lasers can also exert a photothermal effect which can be exploited for coagulation and vaporisation of stones as commonly used in the genitourinary system. Stones can also be broken by using the photomechanical effect of laser, which has been incorporated in intracorporeal intraluminal laser systems. Another important property is the photodynamic or photochemical effect wherein preferentially larger amounts of laser energy is focussed on tissues which uptake photochemical substances like tumours. Short duration pulse lasers can also exert a photoacoustic effect which can be used for management of stones.

Lasers can be used in various modes:

- *Continuous mode*: In this mode the laser is produced and directed continuously with a low power output varying from 1000–5000 W.
- *Pulsed mode*: In the pulsed mode, short duration peaks of laser are directed at a 100-fold higher power.
- *Q switch mode*: Excited photons are directed suddenly producing a very high power output.

The Argon Beam Laser

The argon beam laser was developed in 1962 as a gaseous state laser and has been widely used for its photocoagulative ability. Argon beam laser has a commonly used wavelength of 488 nm and falls in the blue green spectrum of light. Argon is rapidly absorbed by pigments like melanin and haemoglobin which makes it a suitable candidate for controlling bleed. The Argon plasma beam electrocoagulation system is used widely as an important method of coagulation especially in dealing with vascular organs. Directed through an endoscope this system can help ablate early cancers of the gastrointestinal tract and manage acute bleeding from the airways, and the gut.

Argon gas being inert and non toxic is the ideal gas for passing electrosurgical current through it. When current is introduced to a beam of argon laser there is rapid ionisation of the particles. This ionisation takes place at much faster speeds than room air and can act as an effective surgical cautery by forming a link between the cautery and the tissue for transfer of energy.

The Nd:YAG Laser

The Nd:YAG laser crystal is made up of the rare trivalent element neodymium with yttrium aluminium garnet ($Y_3Al_5O_{12}$). Nd:YAG laser took a long time to make its way into medical equipment. This laser has been used in various modes depending upon the characteristics needed. The high power continuous wave operation is used in heavy duty cutting and exploits the thermal lensing phenomenon. The high intensity Q switched operation is more commonly employed in surgical lasers where high power laser is fired as pulses. The Nd:YAG laser can also be used in single mode operation. This laser has a wavelength of 1064 nm and falls under the near infrared spectrum of light. A pointing laser falling in the visible spectrum can be used to guide the Nd:YAG beam.

Nd:YAG laser has a deep penetration of 5–6 mm from the point of contact. It offers excellent haemostasis and causes tumor ablation by coagulative necrosis. This laser has found application in most fields of surgery including ophthalmic surgery, management of endobronchial and other endoluminal tumours, skin lesions, ablation of thyroid, in management of stone disease and prostate growth. It is commonly employed at a setting of 20–30 watts.

The Ho:YAG Laser (Figs 16.1A and B)

The active medium of the Ho:YAG crystal laser is made up of aluminium, yttrium and garnet doped with holmium. Holmium based lasers have found their existence and application in surgical fields in recent times. This laser has a wavelength of 2100 nm, positioning it in the near Infrared spectrum of light. It is also a solid state laser with minimal penetration in tissue, up to a distance of 0.5 mm. It is very well-absorbed in water making it relatively safer to use. In the Q switched mode, the laser is used with pulse duration of 250–350 microseconds and a setting of 0.6–1.2 J at 8–10 Hz which allows precise cutting and tumour ablation.

The laser is widely employed for procedures like dacrorhinocystostomy and lithotripsy. The higher margin of safety has made this laser extremely popular among urologists and its use is employed in vaporising stones, cutting through strictures and ablating prostatic and bladder tissue. The clinical relevance of concern regarding production of cyanide as a by-product of uric acid stone lithotripsy is still undetermined and should be taken while using holmium laser for uria acid stones.

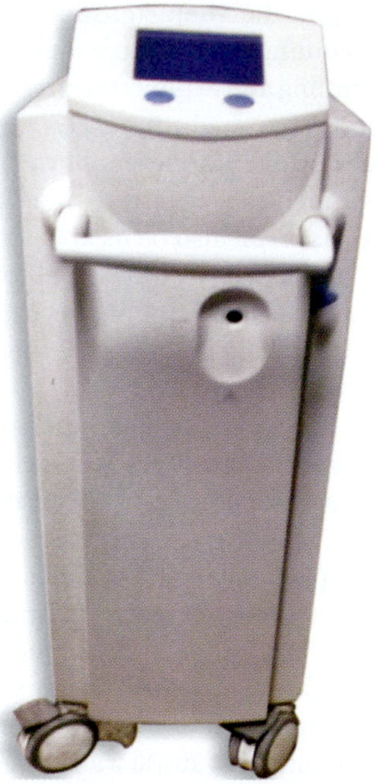

Figure 16.1A: Showing machine of holmium laser

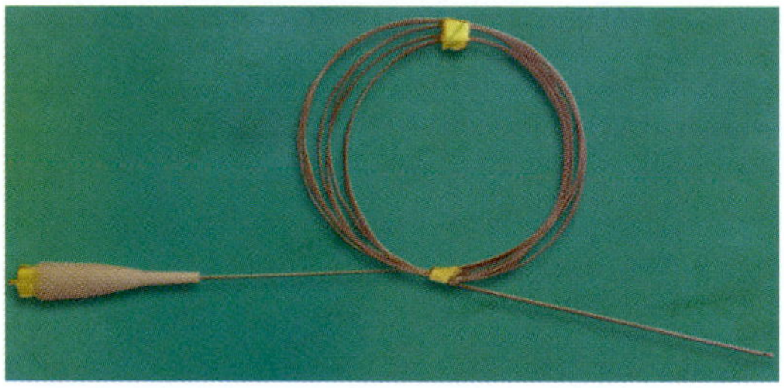

Figure 16.1B: Fibre of holmium laser

The KTP Laser (Fig. 16.2)

The KTP or potassium titanyl phosphate laser is a frequency doubled Nd:YAG beam passing through a KTP crystal. With a wavelength of 532 nm this laser falls in the visible spectrum and emits a green light. The light emitted by the KTP laser is absorbed mainly by haemoglobin, which is protective for the surrounding tissue due to vascular selectivity of this laser. KTP laser causes photoselective vaporisation and desiccation of tissue and has been used in treating endoluminal growths, skin lesions, hypertrophy of the prostate and ocular surgery. These lasers have a greater depth of penetration.

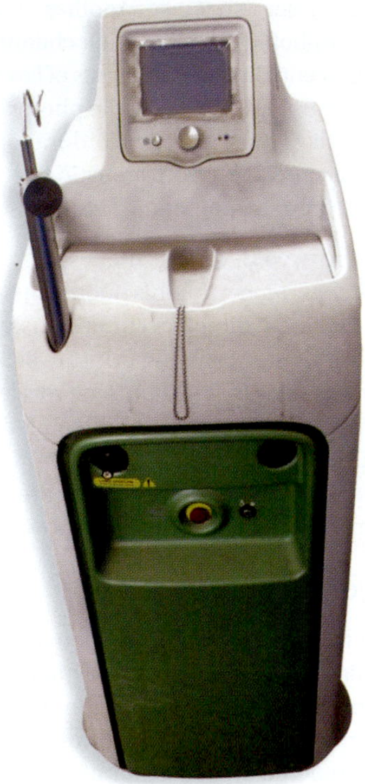

Figure 16.2: Showing KTP laser machine

The Diode Laser

The diode laser is produced by a p-n type of linear array which provides flexibility and portability of use. It employs a small crystal over which substances like indium gallium nitride, aluminium gallium arsenide are doped. These lasers are therefore small and have found use in various fields. Common wavelengths range from 300–3000 nm depending upon the crystal used and the substance doped on the crystal. Diode lasers have a high gain, signifying that they are more efficient compared to other lasers. These lasers can be used in continuous mode as well as in the pulsed mode. Diode lasers have been used for cosmetic surgery, superficial skin tumors, early stage endoluminal lesions in otorhinolaryngology and urology and endovascular surgery.

Carbon Dioxide Laser

The carbon dioxide laser is a 10600 nm laser that falls in the far infrared spectrum and requires visible aiming by a diode laser. It can be used in both continuous and short pulse mode and is considered the gold standard for ablative resurfacing. It can be used in several different gas combinations of CO_2 with helium, and nitrogen. It provides more control over the depth of penetration and can be absorbed by both the intracellular and extracellular water to produce vaporisation. The CO_2 laser is one of the earliest gaseous state lasers to be produced and is a major workhorse in dermatological resurfacing surgery.

Here are some of the various applications of laser in surgery:

- Resurfacing skin and management of keloids and hypertrophic scars
- Management of cutaneous vascular lesions like telangiectasias, hemangiomas, and venous malformations, verious lakes and angiomas
- Cosmetic applications like resurfacing, dermatosis, photoepilation, pigmentation and hypopigmentation, etc.
- Management of malignant and benign skin tumours and inflammatory conditions
- Management of varicose veins in the form of intravenous laser therapy (IVLT)
- Ophthalmic surgery of the cornea, uvea, vitreoretinal and more
- Urological applications like management of stones, BPH and strictures
- Coagulation in surgery of solid vascular viscera
- Photodynamic therapy
- Orthopaedic arthroscopic surgery, meniscal surgery, disc compression, etc.
- Pulmonary and thoracic surgery
- Endoluminal management of polyps, varices and strictures in gastroenterology.

Types of Laser Hazards

1. *Eye:* Acute exposure of the eye to lasers can lead to corneal or retinal burns. Chronic exposure to excessive levels may cause corneal injury, cataracts or retinal injury.
2. *Skin:* Acute exposure to high levels may cause skin burns, while carcinogenesis may occur for ultraviolet wavelengths (290–320 nm).
3. *Chemical:* Some lasers require hazardous or toxic substances to operate (i.e. chemical dye, exciter lasers).
4. *Electrical:* Most lasers utilise high voltages that can be lethal.
5. *Fire:* The solvents used in dye lasers are flammable. High voltage pulse or flash lamps may cause ignition. Flammable materials may be ignited by direct beams or specular reflections from high power continuous wave (CW) infrared lasers.

Lasers and Eyes

Laser light in the visible to near infrared spectrum (i.e. 400–1400 nm) can cause damage to the retina resulting in scotoma (blind spot in the fovea). This wave band is also known as the "retinal hazard region". Laser light in the ultraviolet (290–400 nm) or far infrared (1400–10,600 nm) spectrum can cause damage to the cornea and/or to the lens. Photoacoustic retinal damage may be associated with an audible "pop" at the time of exposure. Visual disorientation due to retinal damage may not be apparent to the operator until considerable thermal damage has occurred.

Symptoms of Laser Eye Injuries

1. Exposure to the invisible ***carbon dioxide laser*** beam (10,600 nm) can be detected by a burning pain at the site of exposure on the cornea or sclera.
2. Exposure to a visible laser beam can be detected by a bright colour flash of the emitted wavelength and an after-image of its complementary colour (e.g. a green 532 nm laser light would produce a green flash followed by a red after-image). *The site of damage depends on the wavelength of the incident or reflected laser beam:* When the retina is affected, there may be difficulty in detecting blue or green colour secondary to cone damage, and pigmentation of the retina may be detected. Exposure to the ***Q-switched Nd:YAG laser*** beam (1064 nm) is especially hazardous and may initially go undetected because the beam is invisible and the retina lacks pain sensory nerves.

Skin Hazards

Exposure of the skin to high power laser beams can cause burns. At the under five watt level, the heat produced from laser will cause a flinch reaction which is a sensation similar to touching any hot object in which one tend to pull hand away or drop it before any major damage occurs. These burns can be quite painful as the affected skin can be cooked, and forms a hard lesion that takes considerable time to heal.

Ultraviolet laser wavelengths may also lead to skin carcinogenesis.

Chemical Hazards

Some materials used in lasers (i.e. excimer, dye and chemical lasers) may be hazardous and/or contain toxic substances. In addition, laser induced reactions can release hazardous particulate and gaseous products.

Electrical Hazards

Lethal electrical hazards may be present in all lasers, particularly in high-power laser systems.

Secondary Hazards including

- Cryogenic coolant hazards
- Excessive noise from very high energy lasers
- Explosions from faulty optical pumps and lamps
- Fire hazards

Laser Safety Standards and Hazard Classification

- Lasers are classified by hazard potential based upon their optical emissions, and necessary control measures are determined by these classifications. In this manner, unnecessary restrictions are not placed on the use of many lasers which are engineered to assure safety.
- In the US, laser classifications are based on American National Standards Institute's (ANSI) Z136.1 safe use of lasers.

ANSI Classifications

- **Class 1** denotes laser or laser systems that do not pose a hazard under normal operating conditions.
- **Class 2** denotes low-power visible lasers or laser systems which do not normally present a hazard, but may present some potential for hazard if viewed directly for extended periods of time.
- **Class 3a** denotes some lasers or laser systems having a CAUTION label that normally would not injure the eye if viewed for only momentary periods (within the aversion response period) with the unaided eye, but may present a greater hazard if viewed using collecting optics. Class 3a lasers have DANGER labels and are capable of exceeding permissible exposure levels. If operated with care Class 3a lasers pose a low risk of injury.
- **Class 3b** denotes lasers or laser systems that can produce a hazard if viewed directly. Normally, Class 3b lasers will not produce a hazardous diffuse reflection.
- **Class 4** denotes lasers or laser systems that produce a hazard not only from reflections, but may also carry significant skin and fire hazards.

General precautions while using lasers:

- Notification in the area where laser is used in the form of warning labels or signboards (Fig. 16.3)
- Safety goggles must be worn at all times to prevent ocular trauma.
- Keep the tip of the optical fibre visible at all times
- Keep the laser in standby mode whenever the fibre is outside the patient's body or is not visible during that part of the procedure.
- Gentle handling of the optical fibre must be done to prevent accidental breakage of the fibre within the scope, to prevent injury to both the patient and the scope.

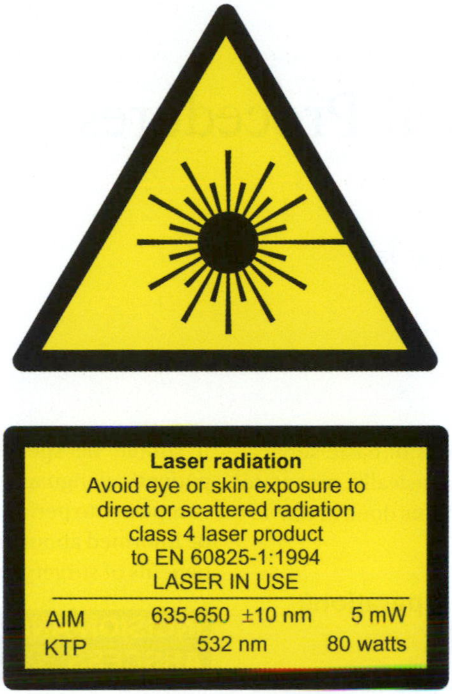

Figure 16.3: Showing display warning regarding laser safety precautions

Laser Protective Eyewear Requirements

1. Laser protective eyewear should be worn by all personnel within the nominal hazard zone (NHZ) of Class 3b and Class 4 lasers where the exposures above the maximum permissible exposure (MPE) occur.
2. Optical density of the laser protective eyewear at each laser wavelength should be notified by the laser safety officer (LSO).
3. All laser protective eyewear should clearly labelled with the optical density and the wavelength for which protection is afforded. This is especially important in areas where multiple lasers are housed.
4. Laser protective eyewear should be inspected for damage prior to use.

Key Points

1. Lasers are commonly used in surgery.
2. All persons using lasers should read the standard operating procedure of that particular laser before using it.
3. Laser operating area should be clearly demarcated.
4. All persons entering that area should use appropriate eye protection device.
5. There should be a laser safety officer to give appropriate training to the staff and to maintain the laser machine.

Basic Surgical Procedures

17

Raman Tanwar, Sudhir Kumar Jain

This chapter describes the steps of basic surgical procedures. This chapter is basically meant to revise the steps of basic operations done in day-to-day practice.

Steps of the Following Operations have been Described

- Incision and drainage of an abscess
- Circumcision
- Intercostal chest tube drainage
- Hydrocele operation
- Appendectomy
- Hernia repair
- Cholecystectomy
- No scalpel vasectomy
- Trendelenburg's operation for varicose veins.

Surgical procedures are an activity requiring careful preoperative workup and dedicated post-operative monitoring. The preoperative workup includes the following:

- Informed consent
- Marking the site to be operated
- Investigations for fitness of the patient for anaesthesia
- Specific investigations pertaining to that surgery.

Informed Consent

Informed consent is the consent given by the patient to undergo a treatment after being fully educated about the advantages and potential harms of the procedure as well as the alternatives. It should be specific for the procedure, in the patient's language, and taken by a surgeon competent to perform procedure. The patient must be informed about the other treatment options, the benefits of surgery and its possible complications.

INCISION AND DRAINAGE OF ABSCESS

Incision and drainage is the primary treatment of an abscess. The procedure is usually performed under local anaesthesia. However the drainage of a large abscess or abscesses that are located deep, abscesses of the breast are preferably performed under general anaesthesia.

Steps

1. The area bearing the abscess is cleaned and draped
2. A field block may be given around the abscess cavity and along the intended line of skin incision. Local anaesthetic injected into the abscess cavity is ineffective.
3. A skin incision is made along Langer's line if possible, or along the longest diameter of the abscess cavity. The skin incision should not extend deep in to the abscess cavity.
4. Further entry is made by thrusting the sinus forceps into the abscess cavity. This method of drainage of abscess is also known as Hilton's method and this avoids injury to underlying neurovascular structures.
5. The jaws are opened and the contents of the abscess cavity are drained.

6. Alternatively, a finger may be inserted into the abscess cavity and all the loculi broken down.
7. The abscess cavity is irrigated with saline and antibiotic solution.
8. Cavity is packed with gauze soaked in antiseptic or iodoform to maintain haemostasis. The pack is removed after 24 hours.
9. A sterile dressing is applied.

DRAINAGE OF BREAST ABSCESS

Breast abscess is an acute, painful condition which may lead to breast tissue destruction. It is a surgical emergency and may discourage breastfeeding. Breast abscess usually results from bacterial mastitis caused by ascending infection by *Staphylococcus aureus.* Drainage or percutaneous needle aspiration is performed if:

1. There is no response to antibiotics in 48 hours.
2. There is persistence of an area of tense induration after completely emptying the breast.
3. Patient is presenting with an area on the breast that is erythematous, warm and fluctuant.

The operation is performed under general anaesthesia, but in case of small abscesses local anaesthesia can be used.

1. The patient lies supine and the breast is cleaned and draped.
2. The incision is placed directly over abscess cavity in a radial direction. The abscess cavity is drained using a long sinus forceps.
3. All loculi inside the abscess cavity should be broken with the tip of sinus forceps or a finger, to prevent any recurrence and to achieve complete drainage.
4. Some large abscesses can be drained through periareolar incision. A drain is placed in the abscess cavity in such cases and brought out through the inframammary fold. The periareolar incision gives a better cosmetic result and minimises scarring. The drain is kept in place by fixing it by safety pin and removed only when drainage subsides.
5. A large abscess cavity on the posterior aspect of breast can be drained through an incision in the inframammary fold.
6. The cavity is thoroughly irrigated with saline and peroxide.
7. The abscess cavity is loosely packed with ribbon gauze.
8. A drain may be left in the dependent portion for drainage of and abscess cavity.
9. If the patient presents with extensive erythema of the overlying skin, a biopsy of the skin should be taken to exclude inflammatory breast cancer.

INTERCOSTAL CHEST TUBE DRAINAGE

Indications

1. Empyema
2. Haemothorax
3. Pneumothorax involving more than 10% of the cavity
4. Tension pneumothorax after stabilisation of patient with needle thoracocentesis
5. Recurrent pneumothorax after repeated aspiration
6. Malignant pleural effusion
7. Surgery with pleural violation, e.g. renal operation through bed of 11th rib.

After taking an informed consent, the patient is made to lie in a supine position with the limb on the affected side in overhead abduction. The procedure is performed under local anaesthesia.

Steps

1. The chest is cleaned and draped.
2. The site for insertion is marked by counting the intercostal spaces from the sternal angle downwards.
3. The site of insertion is marked in the triangle of safety which is bounded by the lateral border of pectoralis major, the mid axillary line and the upper border of the 5th rib.
4. Local anaesthetic agent is infiltrated along the line of incision down to the pleura.
5. A transverse incision is made along the Langer's line in the site marked just above the lower rib of the intercostal space.

6. The incision is developed in layers using artery forceps. Muscles encountered are split until the pleura is reached.
7. The pleura is punctured using a hemostat under vision. Resistance is encountered while puncturing the pleura.
8. A finger is then introduced into the pleural cavity to make sure that lung is not adherent to the chest wall at the proposed site of tube insertion.
9. A chest tube is introduced through the incision, and directed towards the para-vertebral gutter. Tube is directed downwards for fluid drainage and upwards for air.
10. The chest tube is connected to an underwater seal bag, and the movement of the fluid column is ensured.
11. Purse string sutures are applied after ensuring the adequate depth and position of the chest tube. A drain fixing suture is also employed to safeguard the chest tube.
12. A sterile dressing is applied around the chest tube which secures the drain in position.
13. The patient is given clamping instructions and sent for a post drainage check chest radiograph to ensure correct position of the tube.

CIRCUMCISION

Indications

1. Phimosis
2. Recurrent attacks of balanitis
3. Balanitis xerotica obliterans limited to the prepuce
4. Bowens disease confined to prepuce
5. Condyloma acuminata
6. Penile carcinoma confined to prepuce
7. Paraphimosis
8. Preputial trauma, e.g. zipper injury
9. Social or religious reasons
10. Difficulty in intercourse due to tight prepuce.

Circumcision is contraindicated in case of hypospadias and in bleeding disorders.

The procedure is performed under local anaesthesia as an office procedure in some countries. It is performed under general anaesthesia in children.

Steps

1. The prepuce is completely retracted and the glans is thoroughly cleaned.
2. A clean-cut incision with a knife is made through the outer surface of the prepuce at the coronal sulcus down to the Buck's fascia (Fig. 17.1).
3. A second incision is made 5 mm proximal to the coronal sulcus on the inner layer of prepuce (Fig. 17.2).
4. Haemostasis is secured and the frenular artery is secured with a figure of 8 suture (Fig. 17.3).
5. The two layers are held together with the help of forceps.
6. Interrupted sutures of 3-0 chromic catgut or vicryl are used to approximate the two incisions.
7. Soft paraffin gauze dressing is applied.

In children with long prepuce, clamp and cut method is used.

HYDROCELE OPERATION

Indications

1. A large hydrocele causing difficulty in carrying out daily activities
2. Hydrocele associated with symptoms of pain or heaviness

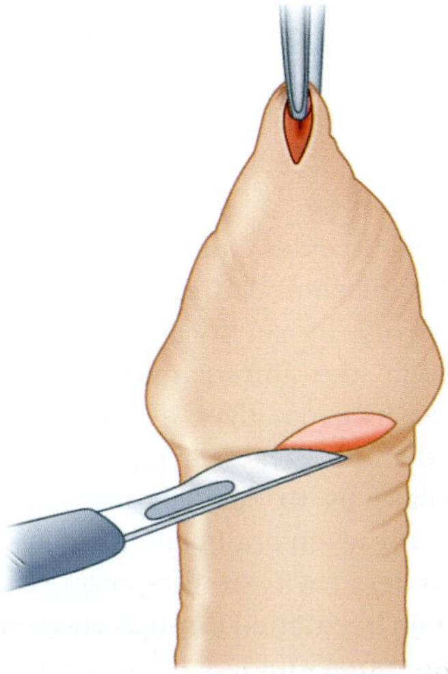

Figure 17.1: Clean incision at coronal sulcus up to Buck's fascia

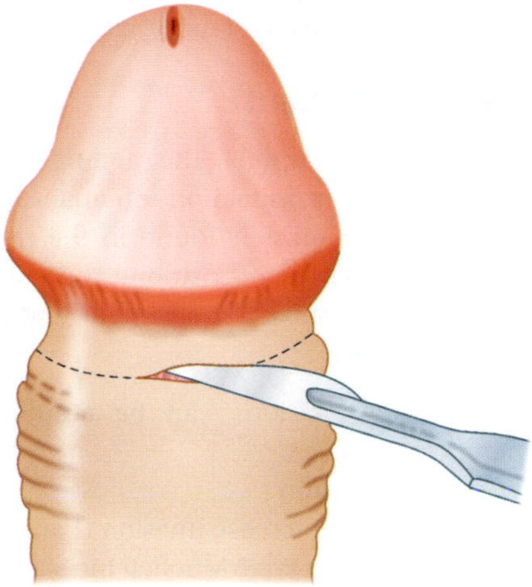

Figure 17.2: Second incision 5 mm proximal to coronal sulcus

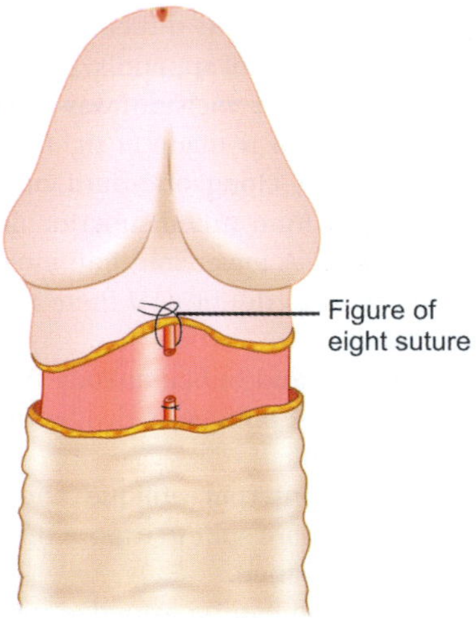

Figure 17.3: Frenular artery secured with figure of 8 suture

3. Difficulty in urination due to burying of the penis in the hydrocele
4. Concern with body image
5. Hydrocele secondary to disease of testis or epididymis
6. Hydrocele prone to repeated trauma.

Surgery for hydrocele can be performed by either the inguinal or the scrotal approach. Scrotal approach is useful in benign hydrocele and is the most common approach utilised.

Steps

1. A vertical or transverse incision is made and developed up to the tunica vaginalis
2. Blunt dissection is performed between the hydrocele sac and the incised layers of the scrotum.
3. Opening is made in the anterior wall of the parietal layer of the tunica and the fluid is sucked out
4. The opening in the tunica is extended both upwards and downwards.
5. If the sac is too large, a part of it is excised and haemostasis secured along the cut margins.
6. The sac is everted and margins of the tunica are sutured using an absorbable catgut suture or vicryl suture.
7. The suturing of the cut margins should be loose enough to permit a finger between the margin and cord structures.
8. The testis is returned back to the scrotum and the scrotal wall is stitched in layers
9. An alternative to the eversion of the sac is plication of the sac or Lord's procedure wherein the hanging curtain of tunica after incision is plicated along the mediastinum of the testis using Vicryl sutures. 8–10 sutures are applied all around the testis after which the complete unit is repositioned back into the scrotum (Fig. 17.4).

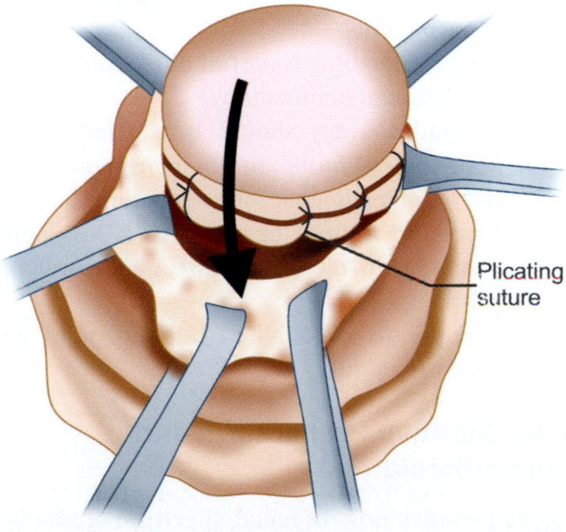

Figure 17.4: Plicating sutures applied and testis reposited back

10. If bleeding is present or in cases of very large hydroceles where extensive blunt dissection is done, a corrugated drain may be placed through a separate stab incision.
11. A scrotal bandage is applied with mild compression to prevent the formation of haematoma and infection.

APPENDICECTOMY

Appendicectomy is the most commonly performed emergency surgical operation around the world.

Indications

1. Acute appendicitis is the most common indication for removing the appendix
2. Interval appendicectomy, 6 weeks after the conservative management of appendicular mass.
3. Patients with recurrent attacks of subacute appendicitis previously known as chronic appendicitis in whom other causes of pain have been ruled out.
4. Mucocele of appendix if detected during abdominal exploration for unrelated pathology.
5. Diverticula containing appendix if detected during course of some other operation.
6. Appendix which is found to contain appendicoliths should be removed because of high chances of future appendicitis in these patients.
7. Appendicectomy is part of Lord's procedure for intestinal malrotation.
8. Appendicectomy should be carried out if appendix is found to be congested after reduction of iliocolic intussuception.
9. Carcinoid tumour of appendix if less than 2 cm, not involving the base, caecal wall or lymph nodes.
10. It appendix is found to be lead point for intussusception.

Preoperative Preparation and Anaesthesia

A preoperative dose of broad-spectrum antibiotic is administered to all patients to cover aerobic and anaerobic organisms. It should be continued if there is significant peritonitis. Spinal anaesthesia or general anaesthesia is employed.

Position of Patient

The patient lies supine. The abdomen should be palpated after induction of anaesthesia. If an appendicular mass is found in the right iliac fossa it is advisable to postpone the surgery in favour of conservative management and interval appendicectomy.

The following incisions can be employed for appendicectomy.

1. Grid iron incision
2. Transverse skin crease incision (Lanz, Rockey Davis or Fowler Weir-Mitchell incision)
3. Lower mid line
4. Rutherford Morrison incision employs cutting of internal oblique and transverses muscle fibres in the line of grid iron skin incision. This is usually done in difficult cases, i.e. retro-caecal position of appendix.

The Grid iron incision was first described by McArthur and is made at right angles to Mc-Burney's, point along one-third of the way on a line drawn from anterosuperior iliac spine to the umbilicus. A lower mid line incision is used if diagnosis is in doubt or if there are features of peritonitis.

- After skin and subcutaneous tissue incision the external oblique is divided in the line of skin incision.
- Fibres of internal oblique and transversus abdominis are split to expose the peritoneum which is opened.
- The incision can be extended medially either by retraction of the rectus muscle or by its division.
- After opening the abdomen the medial end of the wound is elevated by a retractor.
- A finger is placed inside the peritoneal cavity to identify and deliver the appendix.
- If the appendix is not felt in this manner the caecum is held by a moist gauze and delivered into the wound by gradual and gentle side to side motion. The appendix is identified by following the taenia of the caecum.
- A finger is used to hook around the appendix to deliver it in the wound. A Babcock tissue

holding forceps is applied around appendix to hold it without crushing.

- The mesoappendix along with appendicular artery is divided between clamps and ligated until the base of the appendix is clear.
- Once the junction of appendicular base with caecum has been identified appendix is crushed with straight clamp about 3–5 mm away from the caecum and is reapplied 3–5 mm away from initial site of crushing.
- The perceived advantages of crushing the base of appendix are following:
  - The serosa becomes rough and the chances of slipping of ligature become less
  - Crushing inverts the mucosa
  - Crushing blocks the lymphatics thus decreasing the chances of retrograde transmission of infection when appendix is being transected
- The base of the appendix is doubly ligated with a 2-0 absorbable suture (Chromic catgut or Polyglactin) at the crushed site
- Appendix is divided between ligature and clamp (Fig. 17.5)
- Exposed mucosa of appendicular stump is cauterised by a spirit swab more often as a surgical ritual without any evidence of benefit behind this practice.

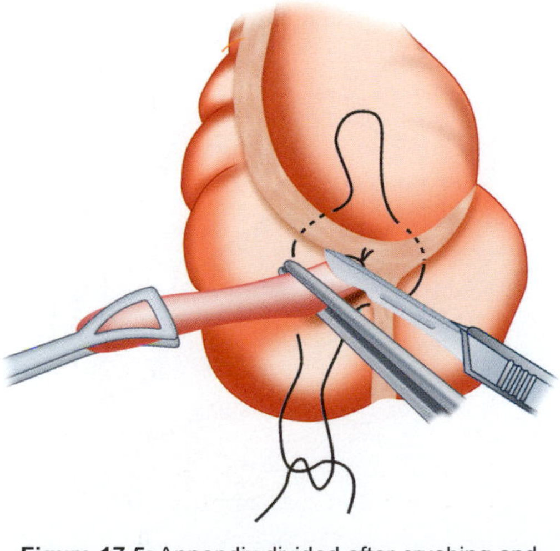

Figure 17.5: Appendix divided after crushing and doubly ligating the base

- The removed appendix along with clamp and the scalpel used to transect the appendix are discarded in a separate kidney dish to minimise contamination.
- Inversion of the appendicular stump is justified only if the base of the appendix is inflamed and cannot be crushed or there is oedema of the appendicular base and there is a fear that ligature may slip.
- Before closure of the wound, peritoneal lavage is done with warm saline.
- It is not necessary to drain the peritoneal cavity in case of nonperforated appendix. However, if there is a localised appendicular abscess or frank purulent fluid, right iliac fossa can be drained through a separate stab incision.
- Wound is closed in layers. Internal oblique and transversus muscles are approximated by an interrupted absorbable 1-0 suture. External oblique is closed by a continuous suture.

TENSION-FREE MESH HERNIOPLASTY

In tension-free hernioplasty the posterior wall of the inguinal canal is strengthened by a prolene mesh 10 × 15 cm in size. As the mesh is placed in between the external oblique aponeurosis and the floor of the inguinal canal, contractions of the external oblique aponeurosis on increasing intra-abdominal pressure (coughing and straining) applies centre pressure over the mesh, thus using intra-abdominal pressure to protect the repair. This operation basically comprises of herniotomy and strengthening of the posterior wall of the inguinal canal by mesh (hernioplasty).

Anaesthesia

Tension free mesh repair can be performed under local, epidural or spinal anaesthesia. Local anaesthesia is preferred for reducible inguinal hernias. For local anaesthesia 1% lignocaine is employed in the dose of 3-4 ml/kg body weight as the maximum dose. For local anaesthesia, infiltration of the local anaesthetic is done in subdermal, intradermal, deep subcutaneous and subaponeurotic planes. A few ml of local anaesthetic is also injected around pubic tubercle, near the neck of the hernial sac and inside the hernial sac, in cases of indirect hernia. Spinal or epidural anaesthesia is employed in cases of large hernias, sliding hernias, irreducible or strangulated hernias or in uncooperative patients.

Position of the Patient

The patient lies supine on the operating table.

- A 5 to 7.5 cm long oblique incision is employed over medial 2/3rd of inguinal ligament starting at the level of pubic tubercle, approximately 2 to 3 cm above it.
- After dividing skin, and subcutaneous tissue, Camper's and Scarpa's fascia are divided in the line of the incision. Superficial external pudendal and superficial inferior epigastric venous tributaries need ligation if encountered.
- External oblique aponeurosis and superficial inguinal ring are exposed and divided in the line of the skin incision to open the inguinal canal. Cut margins of external oblique aponeurosis are held in mosquito artery forceps (Fig. 17.6).
- An upper flap is separated from the underlying internal oblique muscle for a distance of at least one inch so that enough space is created to place a mesh over internal oblique. The iliohypogastric nerve comes into view at this stage, and should be safeguarded.
- Lower flap of external oblique is reflected downward till one sees the inturned portion of the inguinal ligament.
- The cord is lifted from the floor of the inguinal canal at the pubic tubercle and the cremasteric fascia and muscle are divided along the whole length of the cord to expose the underlying sac.
- Cremastric artery and vein usually need ligation or cauterisation near the deep ring.
- Indirect sac is anterolateral to the vas deferens and spermatic vessels and is separated from them up to the neck of the sac. An indirect sac can be ligated at the neck and the remaining portion excised or pushed back into the peritoneal cavity (Fig. 17.7).
- Direct hernial sacs which are posteromedial to the cord are simply pushed back into the peritoneal cavity.
- If the sac is large, it is inverted with absorbable sutures.
- Strengthening of the posterior wall of the inguinal canal is performed by polypropylene mesh measuring 10 by 15 cm.

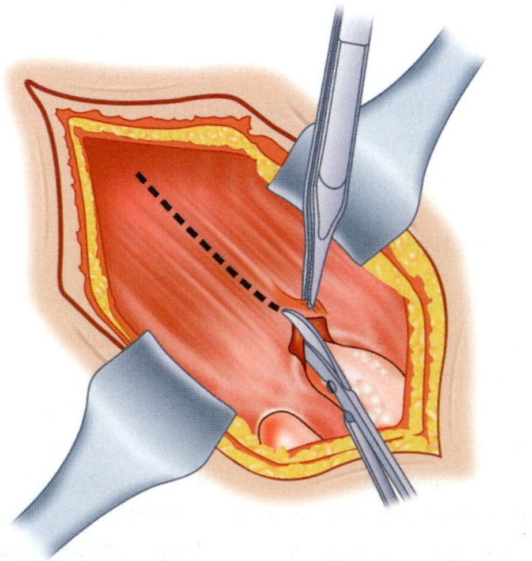

Figure 17.6: Aponeurosis of external oblique muscle incised

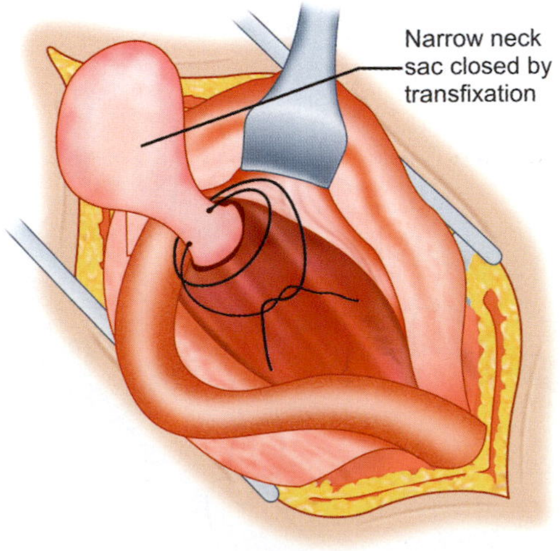

Figure 17.7: Sac isolated and neck closed by transfixation

- The medial border of the mesh is rounded to correspond to the shape of medial corner of the inguinal canal and is overlapped at least by 1 × 1.5 cm over the rectus sheath and sutured to it by prolene 2-0 sutures.
- Lower border of the mesh is sutured to the inturned portion of the inguinal ligament by continuous 2-0 prolene sutures upto the level of the deep ring.
- A slit is made at the lateral end of the mesh creating two tails, upper wide (2/3rd) and lower narrower (1/3rd). Two tails of the mesh are overlapped to contain the spermatic cord and the lower margins of both are stitched to the inguinal ligament. Crossing of the two tails creates an internal ring.
- The upper margin of the mesh is fixed to underlying internal oblique by means of interrupted sutures.
- The mesh should be lax, tented up or slightly wrinkled rather than lying flat to avoid tension on mesh when the patient stands and the fascia transversalis is pushed forwards. Medially the mesh should lay 1.5 to 2 cm medial to the pubic tubercle, with the upper margin of the mesh 3–4 cm above the Hesselbach's triangle and 3–4 cm lateral to the deep ring (Fig. 17.8).
- The external oblique aponeurosis is stitched by continuous prolene 1-0 sutures.
- Skin and subcutaneous tissue are closed and sterile surgical dressing applied.

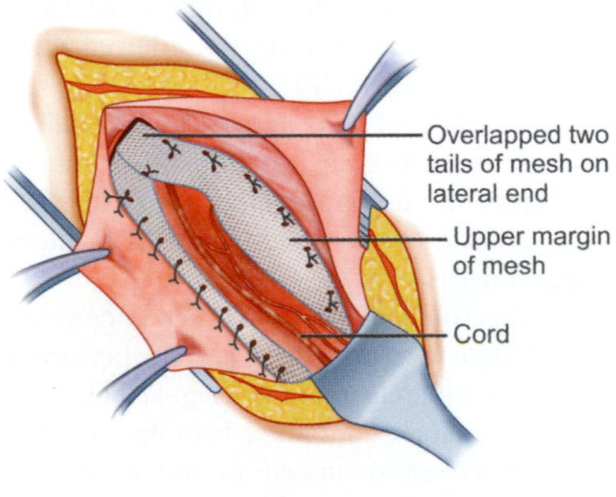

Figure 17.8: Mesh placed on the posterior wall

Herniorrhaphy

In the era of modern surgical practice tissue repair might be indicated in the following situations:

1. In cases of strangulated inguinal hernia where bowel resection is carried out, mesh hernioplasty is contraindicated because of high chances of mesh infection.
2. If the patient has a known allergy to mesh material.
3. If the patient refuses to have foreign material implantation in his or her body.
4. There are reports that in young males in the reproductive age with bilateral groin hernia, mesh repair on both sides may produce oligospermia or subfertility because of entrapment of vas in the mesh. Synthetic mesh, e.g. prolene mesh commonly used in hernia repair can cause an intense inflammatory response leading to obstruction or narrowing of the vas. Prolene mesh in the young male especially if bilateral hernia repair is needed should be used with caution. Other alternatives such as tissue repair or laparoscopic repair might be a better option.

The following tissue repairs are most popular:

1. Bassini's repair
2. Marcy repair
3. Iliopubic tract repair
4. McVay repair
5. Shouldice repair

Bassini's repair and shouldice repair are most commonly performed and described below.

Anaesthesia

The majority of open groin hernia repairs can be performed under local anaesthesia unless the hernia is very big, sliding or inguinoscrotal. Commonly used agents for local anaesthesia are 0.5–1% lignocaine with epinephrine or 0.25% bupivacaine with epinephrine or a combination of both. Sodium bicarbonate can be added in the solution to alter the pH, which is thought to decrease the pain of injection.

10 ml of this preformed solution is injected just medial to the anterosuperior iliac spine in a fan-shaped manner to block the ilioinguinal and iliohypogastric nerves. Another 60 ml

is injected as a field block along the line of the proposed incision in the intradermal, subcutaneous and subaponeurotic planes. After opening the inguinal canal 5-10 ml is injected around the neck of hernia sac, and a few ml is instilled inside the hernial sac. Five to ten ml of the solution is also injected around the pubic tubercle to block the genital branch of the genitofemoral nerve.

Common Steps

Classically, an oblique skin incision is placed 2 cm above and parallel to the inguinal ligament over its medial 2/3rd.

The incision is deepened through the Camper's and Scarpa's fascia till external oblique aponeurosis is exposed.

External oblique aponeurosis is incised in the line of incision through superficial inguinal ring.

After opening the inguinal canal, upper flap of the external oblique aponeurosis is separated from underlying internal oblique and rectus muscle by blunt dissection. Iliohypogastric nerve is identified and safeguarded. Inferior flap is reflected down till the shelving edge of the inguinal ligament is seen.

Margins of the superior and inferior flaps of external oblique are held in artery forceps. Cord structures are lifted up away from the floor of the inguinal canal by blunt dissection near the pubic tubercle. After lifting the cord structures they are held in an umbilical tape or in a penrose drain.

Cremastric muscle is divided along the whole length of the cord to expose the underlying structures. The hernial sac is isolated from remaining cord structures till the neck of sac (Fig. 17.9).

Once the sac has been isolated from cord structures it is opened at the fundus to make sure that all contents have been reduced. Sac can either be reduced in the preperitoneal space without excision or sac can be ligated at neck by transfixation and remaining part of the sac excised. If the hernia sac is complete and reaching up to the scrotum there is no need to isolate it completely, rather it can be divided midway and distal part of the sac can be left *in situ* along with cord structures after laying it open on its anterior wall.

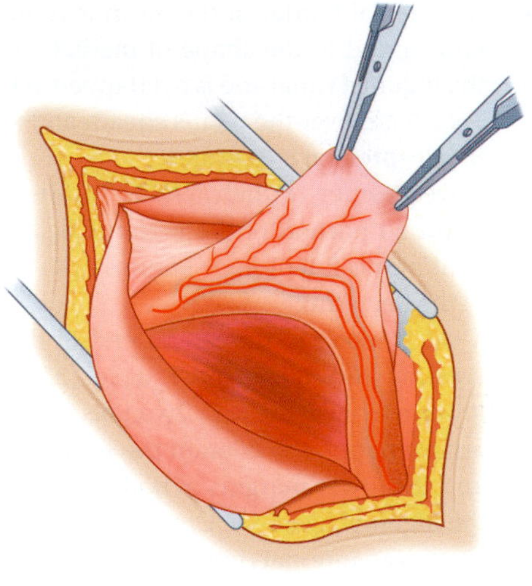

Figure 17.9: Hernial sac being isolated from rest of the cord structures

Laying open of the distal remaining sac prevents the future hydrocele formation.

BASSINI'S REPAIR

Edwards Bassini advocated high ligation of the sac with reconstruction of posterior wall of the inguinal canal. Bassini emphasised the incision in the external oblique aponeurosis superior to skin incision so that suture line of the repair does not lie in line with the line of closure of the external oblique.

After handling the hernial sac fascia transversalis is opened from the internal ring to pubic tubercle (Fig. 17.10).

Upper flap of the fascia transversalis is dissected upwards away from the preperitoneum, thus creating a flap comprising of fascia transversalis, transversus abdominis and internal oblique muscle.

The first stitch in the Bassini's repair consists of a flap of triple layer superiorly and the periosteum of the pubic tubercle inferiorly (Fig. 17.11).

Repair is then continued laterally and triple layer flap is approximated to the reflected in turned portion of the inguinal ligament by means of interrupted sutures. Sutures are continued till the medial edge of the deep ring. Six to eight

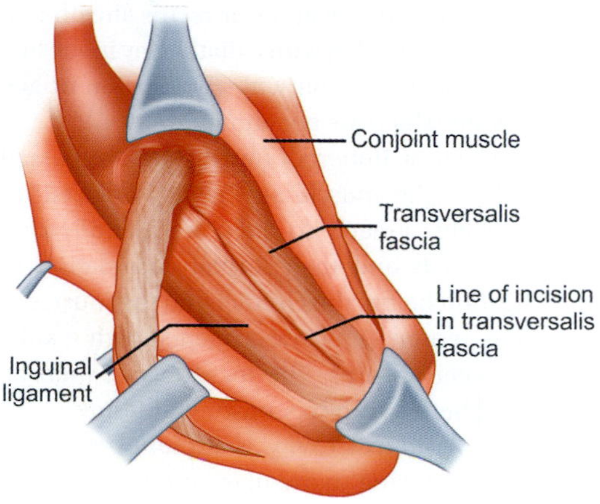

Figure 17.10: Fascia transversalis opened

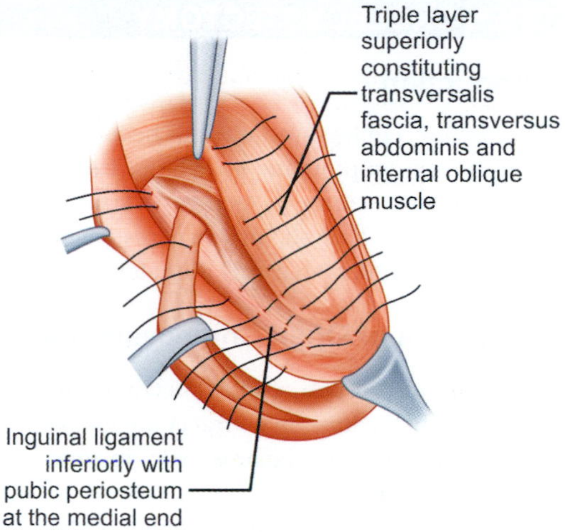

Figure 17.11: Performing the Bassini's repair

stitches are used to approximate the triple layer to the in turned portion of the inguinal ligament.

Original Bassini's repair has been modified in North America where fascia transversalis is not incised. Only internal oblique and transversus abdominis muscles are approximated to the inguinal ligament.

SHOULDICE REPAIR

This repair, popularised by Shouldice Hospital, is also known as double breasting the inguinal canal. It principally involves reinforcing the floor of the inguinal canal by a four layered repair.

After the inguinal canal is opened in the usual manner described above, the transversalis fascia is then split in its middle, starting from the deep ring till the pubis, so that it forms a superior and an inferior flap, which are also dissected free from the pro-peritoneal fat.

The repair begins with a continuous suture of non-absorbable material that starts from the pubic tubercle, and approximates the free edge of the lower flap of transversalis fascia to the lateral border of the rectus medially and the undersurface of the upper flap of trasversalis fascia laterally, leaving a free edge to the latter.

After reaching the deep ring, the suture returns from lateral to medial as the second layer, picking up the free edge of the upper flap of trasversalis fascia and approximating it to the inguinal ligament all the way to the pubic tubercle.

A second length of the suture is now taken, starting at the deep ring laterally, and continuing medially as the third layer, approximating the internal oblique and tranversus abdominis superiorly to the inner aspect of the external oblique aponeurosis, just adjacent to the inguinal ligament.

This suture then reverses after reaching the pubic tubercle as the fourth layer, travelling laterally to the deep ring, again approximating the internal oblique and tranversus abdominis superiorly to the inner aspect of the external oblique aponeurosis in a more superficial plane.

The repair thus creates four layered reinforcement of the floor of the inguinal canal, the adjacent layers being created in a double-breasted manner. After the repair of the floor of the inguinal canal using one of the methods described above, the canal is closed by suturing the flaps of the external oblique aponeurosis using a continuous nonabsorbable suture.

OPEN CHOLECYSTECTOMY

Introduction

Laparoscopic cholecystectomy has become a gold standard for symptomatic gallstone disease and open cholecystectomy is being performed less often these days limited, only to cases where safe laparoscopic cholecystectomy is not feasible.

Indications of Open Cholecystectomy

Indications for open cholecystectomy in the present era of laparoscopic surgery are following:

1. Conversion from laparoscopic to open in following situations:
   a. Elective conversion to open if there is anatomical obscuration in cholecysto-hepatic triangle with risk of injury to adjacent structures.
   b. Forced conversion if there is an injury to common bile duct or duodenum or if there is bleeding which cannot be controlled by laparoscopic means.
   c. Patient unwilling for laparoscopic surgery.
   d. Patient with chronic obstructive airway disease increasing the chances of CO_2 toxicity.
   e. Patient suffering from severe cardiac disease with low ejection fraction.
   f. Gallstones associated with portal hypertension.
   g. Gallstones associated with cirrhosis
   h. Refractory coagulopathy in which laparoscopic surgery should be avoided.
   i. Empyema of gallbladder.
   j. Emphysematous cholecystitis.
   k. Perforation of gallbladder or pericholecystic abscess.
   l. Cholecystoenteric fistula.
   m. Multiple past upper abdominal surgeries.
2. Carcinoma gallbladder

Steps

1. The subcostal incision is placed 4 cm below and parallel to the right costal margin and usually extends from close to the midline to the tip of ninth costal cartilage.
2. Once the skin and subcutaneous tissue have been incised, the anterior rectus sheath and muscle is divided with a diathermy in the line of the skin incision with coagulation of any vessels which are encountered.
3. A Mayo or Roberts's forceps can be passed behind the muscle so that it is placed on a slight streach to help in identification of vessels and their formal coagulation or ligation before they retract into the muscle.
4. The peritoneum is next opened with a knife between forceps. The incision can then be lengthened with scissors or diathermy.
5. The peritoneal cavity is explored systematically paying particular attention to the stomach, duodenum, liver, gallbladder, small bowel and colon.
6. The right hand is passed over the liver to break the vacuum and to introduce air so that the liver can descend into the wound. The gallbladder is grasped with two pairs of sponge-holding forceps, one pair being applied to the fundus and the other to Hartmann's pouch.
7. The gallbladder is retracted downwards, outwards and laterally. Any adherent structure with gallbladder which is generally omentum or colon or duodenum is carefully separated using combination of blunt and sharp dissection.
8. Two moist packs are then inserted. The first pack retracts the colon downwards and prevents bowel from entering the operative field. The second is placed so that the duodenum, stomach and free edge of the lesser omentum can be retracted to the left throughout the operation. These packs can be kept in place by Deaver's retractors held by assistants or by assistant hands.
9. The anterior layer of peritoneum overlying the hepatoduodenal ligament is then incised near the region of neck of gallbladder using dissecting scissors (Fig. 17.12).
10. Dissection is carried out in cholecystohepatic triangle using right angle dissection forceps or a pledget held in a pair of Mayo or Robert's forceps. The anatomy of the biliary tree is assessed carefully, noting the diameter of the

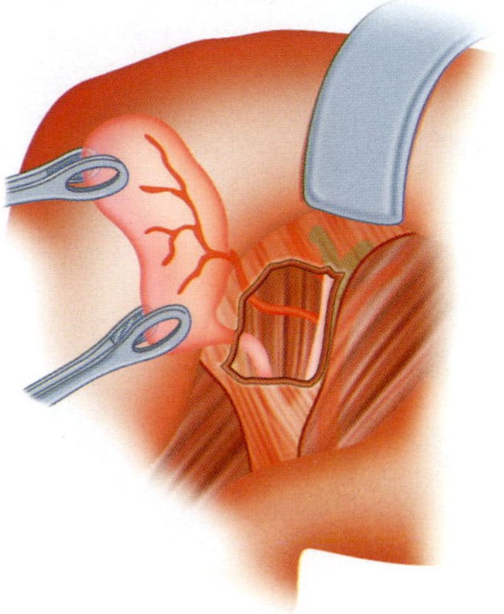

Figure 17.12: Placing the packs and retractors and incising the anterior layer of peritoneum over Calot's triangle

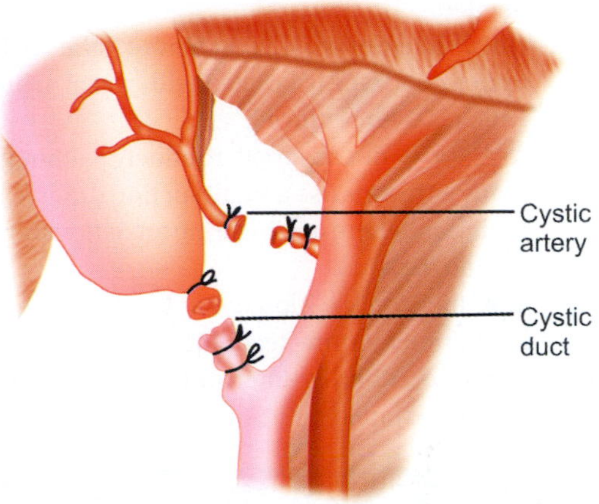

Figure 17.13: Cystic duct and artery ligated and divided

cystic duct and common hepatic/common bile duct.

11. The right angle dissection forceps are used to sweep adventitial tissues carefully away from the cystic duct and to display the triangle bounded by the cystic duct, common hepatic duct and inferior edge of the liver. This manoeuvre usually brings the cystic artery into view.
12. The cystic duct is securely tied with polyglactin or silk suture. Two sutures are applied on common bile duct side and one on the gallbladder side.
13. The cystic artery is also doubly ligated and both structures are then divided (Fig. 17.13).
14. The gallbladder is kept under tension by gentle traction from the surgeon's left hand, and the fold of peritoneum attaching the gallbladder to the liver is divided using a combination of sharp dissection and electrocoagulation (Fig. 17.14).
15. On occasion, it may be safer to remove the gallbladder using a 'fundus first' approach, particularly when inflammation or adhesion formation makes it difficult to display the common bile duct, cystic duct and cystic artery.

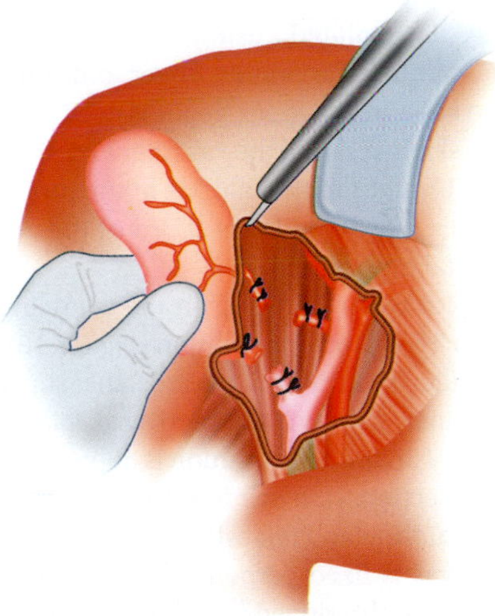

Figure 17.14: Fold of peritoneum between gallbladder and liver divided

16. Regardless of whether the gallbladder is removed fundus first or by the more conventional method, a small swab is placed in the gallbladder bed to control oozing.
17. Any small bleeding vessels are coagulated, and if bleeding is troublesome and persists, a gauze swab or small pack is left in the gallbladder bed for 3–5 min.
18. If this does not produce adequate haemostasis, underrunning of the bleeding

points with a fine absorbable suture may be needed.

19. Once haemostasis is achieved, the right upper quadrant is lavaged with warm saline which is then removed.
20. A drain is not inserted routinely, although many surgeons use a small suction drain (e.g. Redivac) if there are lingering anxieties about haemostasis.
21. The incision is closed in layers using a continuous suture technique, and the skin is closed either by interrupted silk or nylon suture or stapler.

NO SCALPEL VASECTOMY

No scalpel vasectomy is a minimally invasive approach to permanent sterilisation of males. It is usually performed in the supine position under local anaesthesia as on an out patient basis.

1. Vas is isolated using the three finger technique. The middle finger and thumb fix the vas and the index finger is used to stretch the skin overlying the vas (Fig. 17.15).
2. It is brought to the midline at the junction of upper 1/3rd and lower 2/3rd of the anterior scrotal raphe.
3. A 1 cm wheal is raised on the overlying skin with 2% lignocaine solution (Fig. 17.16).
4. Needle is advanced towards the superficial inguinal ring in the perivasal plane and 2 ml of anaesthetic solution is deposited.
5. The second side vas is similarly brought to the midline and anaesthetised.
6. The vas is fixed perpendicular to the line of the vas with a ringed clamp or extracutaneous vas fixation forceps.
7. The vas dissecting forceps is inserted into the lumen of the vas.
8. The forceps is gently opened and all the overlying layers separated until vas is exposed.
9. The vas is grasped between the blades of the dissection forceps and the wrist is supinated. The vas is thus delivered out of the wound. The ringed clamp is released simultaneously.
10. The vascular structures and fascia surrounding the vas are stripped using the vas dissection forceps.

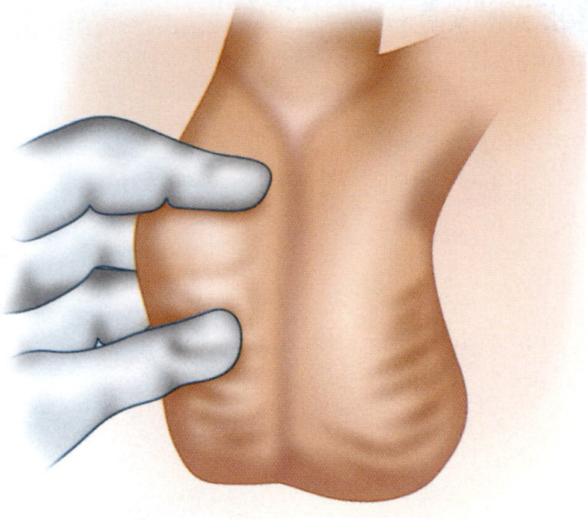

Figure 17.15: Vas isolated using 3 finger technique

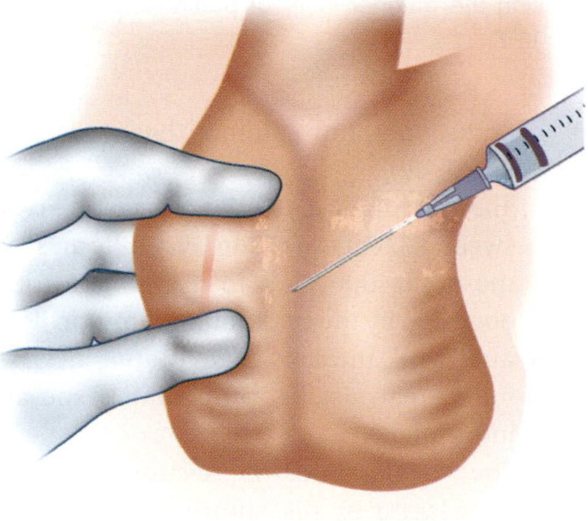

Figure 17.16: Wheal raised over the overlying skin

11. The ends of the vas are ligated and a 1 cm segment is removed. The ligature on the abdominal end is kept long.
12. The cut ends are deposited back and the abdominal end is brought up again by pulling the tie attached to it.
13. The re-emerging end is enclosed in fascia around which another tie is taken for fascial interpositioning.
14. The other side is similarly operated through the same wound.
15. An antiseptic dressing is applied on the midline wound.

TRENDELENBURG'S OPERATION FOR VARICOSE VEINS

The Trendelenburg's operation is performed for saphenofemoral valve incompetence leading to varicose veins. It is done in the supine position under spinal or general anaesthesia.

Position of Patient

1. Patient lies supine with the table tilted head down to an angle of 15°.
2. A 7–8 cm long oblique incision centred over anatomical marking of saphenous, i.e. 3.75 cm below and lateral to pubic tubercle is made parallel to the fold of the groin.
3. Incision is carried deeper till the superficial fascia is seen, which is then incised. Gauze dissection can be used to separate the fat and exposes the saphenofemoral junction. Saphena magna is dissected gently using a Mayo's tissue cutting scissors.
4. Femoral vein is exposed 1 cm above and below the saphenofemoral junction.
5. The all tributaries joining the termination of saphenous vein are defined and ligated.
6. The end of the long saphenous vein is flush ligated at saphenofemoral junction with silk and a second ligature is used to transfix the junction to avoid slipping of ligature (Fig. 17.17).
7. Femoral vein is inspected above and below the junction and long saphenous vein divided.
8. Stripping of the long saphenous vein is performed up to a level just below knee joint.
9. Incision is closed in layers.

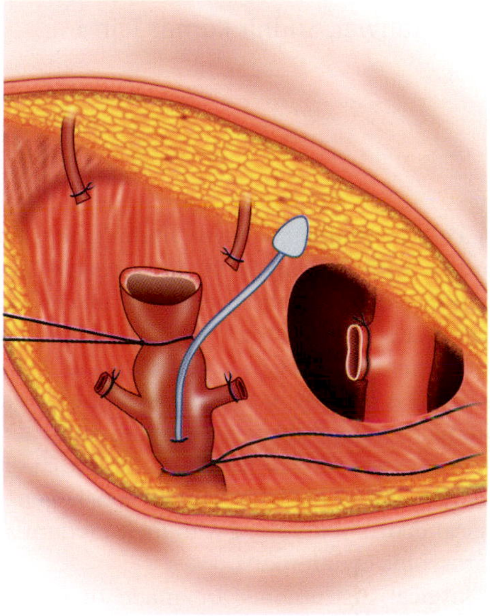

Figure 17.17: Long saphenous vein flush ligated at saphenofemoral junction

General Surgical Instruments

18

Raman Tanwar, Sudhir Kumar Jain

Surgical instruments have undergone rapid changes with advances in technology. These advances include discovery of newer and better materials, minimal ways of access, and development of gadgets to handle and dissect tissues. This has led to expansion of the surgical armamentarium, which a surgical student or trainee is expected to be familiar with. This chapter aims to introduce the conventional general surgical instruments along with their modern and laparoscopic counterparts.

Surgical instruments are made of stainless steel alloys with different grades (most common is 304) and properties. These alloys are inert, resilient and allow construction of sharp edges. However during surgery they can get heated up or can conduct electricity and also can reflect the glare of OT lighting system upon the operating surgeon if not used with proper etiquette. Other problems with stainless steel alloys include poor galling resistance, loss of the sharpness of edges and wear/tear on repeated use. Although stainless steel is relatively resistant to rusting its durability is increased by a process called passivation which is an engineering or physical chemistry process which makes the material passive to the effects of environmental factors such as air or water. During passivation a light layer of metal oxide is coated over the equipment.

Stainless steel equipments are durable if cared for properly. They tend to lose sharpness with passage of time but their exterior can be maintained if cleaned regularly. Most hospitals have a specific protocol for the care of their equipment. This protocol usually involves the following steps:

1. Thorough cleaning with tap water to remove gross contamination
2. Gross inspection and care of left over soiling, misalignment, loose screws or joints, roughness, dullness, gross physical damage, staining or corrosion.
3. Soap/detergent based cleaning of grease and body fluids
4. Deionised water is used for last round of cleaning
5. Ultrasonic cleaning by cavitation (if available) for adherent tissue fat.

   Following the cleaning process instruments can be sterilised by one of the following methods:

   a. By autoclave
   b. Orthoparaldehyde (OPA)
   c. Gluteraldehyde
   d. Ethylene oxide
   e. Formalin.

Storage of Instruments

Instruments in bulk are kept in ramps and trays like the DIN Tray or OP wash Cart. Small or single instruments are kept in cassettes or peel pouches for sterilisation. Mesh trays can be used for cleaning and sterilising small detachable and reusable parts. It is advised that all jaws be opened before cleaning. Towels are used to separate instruments, with the larger ones kept below the smaller instruments. Tips of all instruments must be aligned in the same direction to avoid damage.

The operating room personnel are usually proficient at defining set of instruments for a particular procedure. Most operating rooms have a set of instruments predefined for upcoming cases, e.g. there would be a laparotomy set, or a laparoscopic cholecystectomy set and a gastrectomy set. These sets will have multiples of all the commonly required instruments for that particular procedure. This is one of the most convenient ways of organising instruments and also makes possible, customisation from a common pool of instruments after the elective surgery list has been posted.

SECTION 1: GENERAL SURGICAL INSTRUMENTS

General surgical handheld instruments can be conveniently classified into:

1. Forceps
   a. Tissue holding forceps: For surgical dissection
   b. Haemostatic forceps: For control of bleeding vessels
   c. Thumb forceps: For holding and dissection
2. Needle holders
3. Retractors
4. Sharps: Needles, trocars and blades
5. Scissors
   a. Tissue cutting: Employed for dividing tissue
   b. Material/Suture cutting: Employed for cutting sutures, dressing, plaster cast, etc.
6. Others: Probes, blade handles, etc.

Tissue Holding Forceps

Tissue holding forceps are the most frequently used surgical instruments which can be used

a. For traction,
b. For retraction,
c. Holding tissues
d. Occasionally for dissection.

They consist of ring handles, shafts converging at a box or screw joint which acts as a fulcrum and the working ends which have tips designed for specific functions. Common examples of tissue holding forceps are Kocher's forceps, Lahey's forceps, Mixters forceps, Rochester-Pean clamp, etc.

Haemostatic Forceps

Haemostatic forceps are used:

a. For achieving control over bleeding vessels
b. Sometimes to hold tough tissue.

The advantage with haemostatic forceps is the high shaft to working end ratio which magnifies the force applied at the rings to about 3–5 times and is utilised in achieving a good and sometimes destructive force. Haemostatic forceps that are commonly used include the mosquito forceps (Fig. 18.1), Robert's artery forceps, Kelly's forceps, Bulldog clamp, Satinsky forceps, etc.

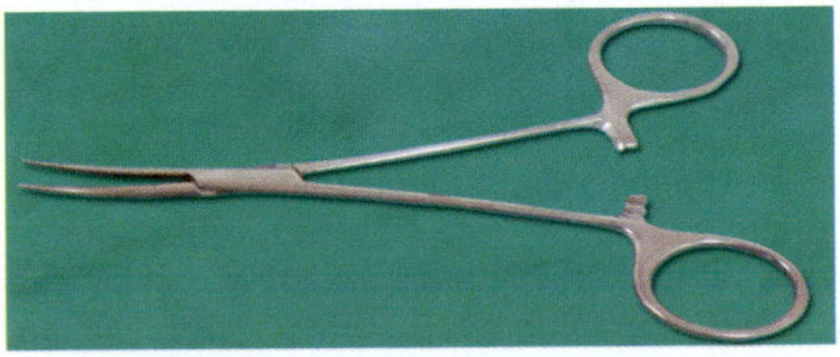

Figure 18.1: Showing mosquito artery forceps

Thumb Forceps

The thumb forceps aid in dissection and tying sutures by holding the tissue and performing retraction using the left hand while the right hand does the dissection or suturing actively. The thumb forceps consists of 4 parts; the tip, shafts handle and a spring joint at the end. Thumb forceps have their tips designed specifically according to their use. They can be simple, serrated, toothed, or pointed for fine dissection. Russian tissue forceps have a cup and surrounding spike/serrations at the working end, designed specifically to dissect the biopsy specimen. Thumb forceps are available in a variety of sizes making tissues at all possible depths accessible. Commonly used thumb forceps are the Adson's pickups, Toothed dissecting forceps, DeBakey's forceps, St Martin forceps.

Needle Holders

Needle holders are designed with a very high mechanical advantage. The working tip is placed very close to the box joint, and the ringed handles are placed quite far such that a force 8–10 times of that applied at the handles is transmitted to the

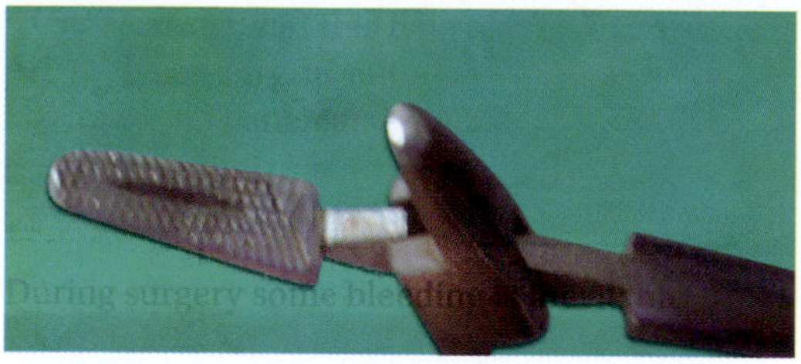

Figure 18.2: Showing tip of needle holder with crisscross serrations and a small pit in the centre

needle holding tip due to fulcrum effects. This along with the multiple striations and a small pit, holds the suture needle firmly. Mayo Hegars is the most commonly used needle holder (Fig. 18.2).

Other needle holders that are used include the Hegar-Baumgartner needle holder, Crile-Wood needle holder, Halsey needle holder, Webster needle holder and the Olsen-Hegar needle holder which is a combined scissors and needle holding forceps. Apart from the regular ringed needle holders with a lock, spring action needle holders like the Kalt needle holder, Paton needle holder, Castroviejo needle holder and the McPherson needle holder are also used, more commonly in the microsurgery or other surgical subspecialties.

Retractors

Compared to the era where fingers and hands were used for retraction, modern day retractors provide a more ergonomic environment letting the assistant work more actively in helping the operating surgeon. Retractors have been classically divided into self-retaining and non-self-retaining retractors. They can also be divided on whether they have blades on one side or both the sides. While the self-retaining retractors avoid the need of an assistant, they also help immensely by reducing surgical fatigue and providing a better field of view compared to the hand. Commonly employed self retaining retractors include the Jolle's thyroid retractor, Balfour self-retaining retractor, Goldstein retractor, Agricola retractor, Barraquer retractor, Davis retractor, McKinney retractor, etc. The non-self-retaining retractors are usually lighter in weight and more ergonomic in design. They may have fenestrations to make the instrument light weight and grips to make it easy to hold. Non-self-retaining retractors include the Czerny's retractor, Langenback's retractor, Rake retractor, Doyens retractor and the Deaver's retractor (Figs 18.3 to 18.6).

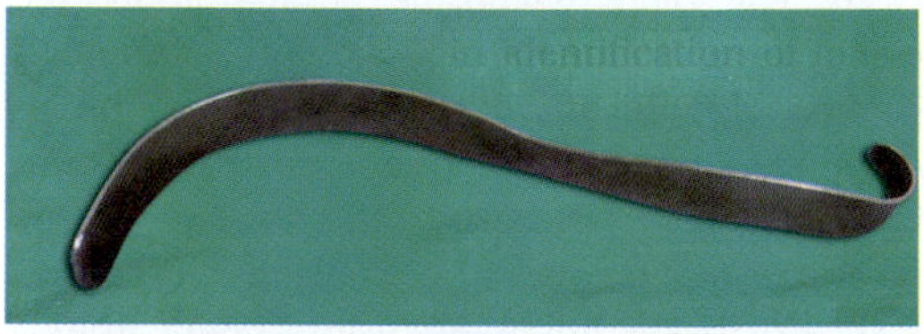

Figure 18.3: Deaver's retractor

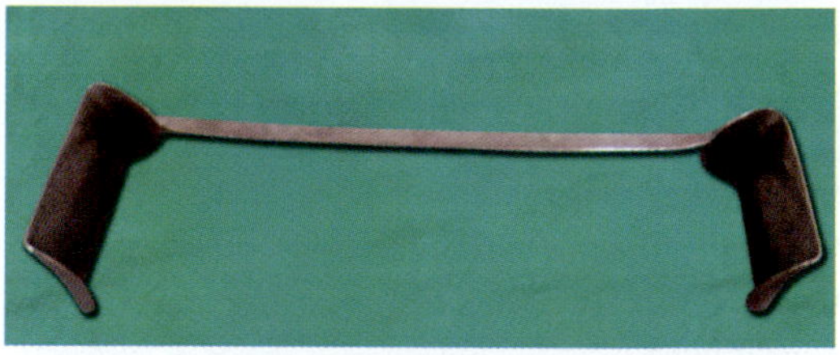

Figure 18.4: Morris retractor

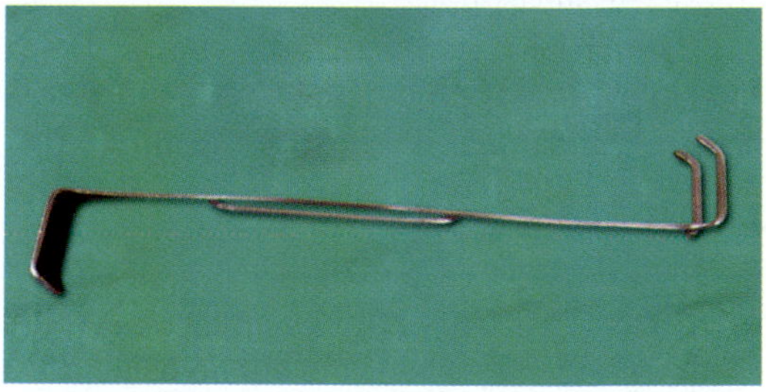

Figure 18.5: Czerny's retractor

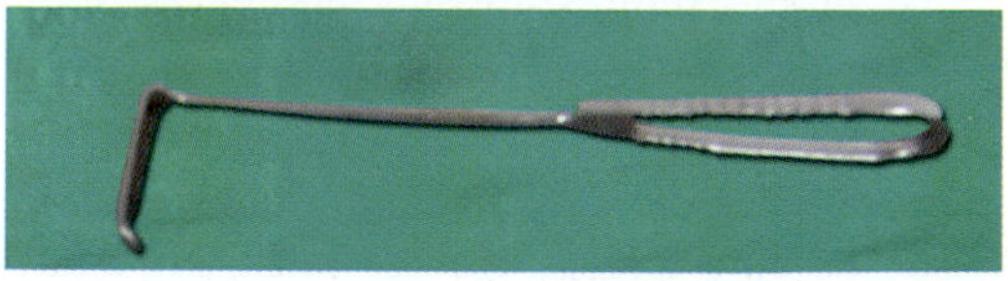

Figure 18.6: Langenbeck's retractor

Scissors

A wide variety of scissors are available to the surgeons with a constant influx of new innovations. Scissors have been modified to suit various fields of surgery. Scissors can be grossly divided as tissue cutting and non tissue cutting. It is essential that scissors used for tissue cutting be sharp and therefore it is best to avoid cutting any other material with them. Tissue cutting scissors are either curved or straight bladed. They may have a screw or a box joint. Nontissue cutting scissors like the gauze cutting, suture cutting or the plaster cutting scissors have their blades modified according to function. Scissors used in microsurgery, ophthalmic surgery and other surgical subspecialities may have spring handles for a finer pincer control.

McGannon Skin Hook (Fig. 18.7)

Skin hook is useful in lifting the skin in procedures of the subcutaneous tissue such as in modified radical mastectomy. It is usually held at right angles to the surface to provide traction.

Backhaus Towel Clip (Fig. 18.8)

Backhaus towel clips are utilised to hold drapes in place while draping the patient to keep only the area of interest along with the bony landmarks exposed. As an alternate, Jones Cross Action towel clips are also frequently used in many centres.

Towels clips have the following uses:

- Used to hold the drapes together at the points of intersection.
- Can be used to lift umbilical pillar during the creation of pneumoperitoneum by open method

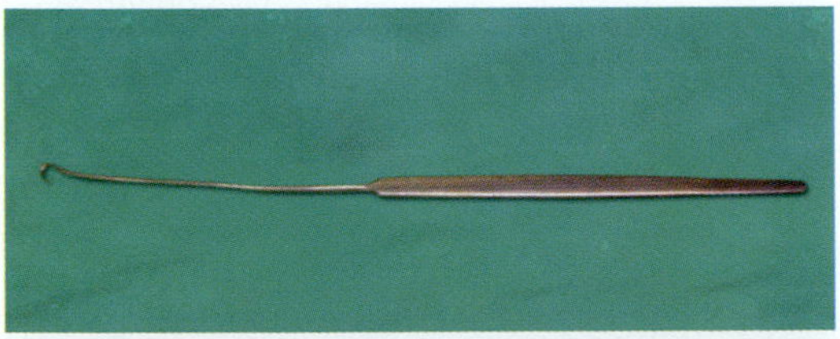

Figure 18.7: McGannon skin hook

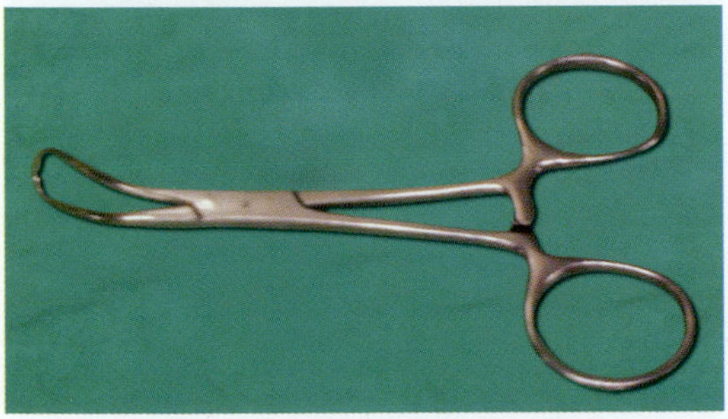

Figure 18.8: Backhaus towel clip

- Used to fix the cables and tubes during laparoscopic procedures.

Lahey's Right Angled Forceps (Fig. 18.9)

Lahey's right angled forceps are used during surgical dissection and haemostasis as described in the earlier sections of this book. They are frequently used for passing sutures in deeper regions as tip can be easily kept under vision avoiding injury to the deeper structures which may not be well visualised.They are also used sometimes to hold a peanut swab.

Longer variants of the Lahey's right angled forceps (20 cm) are commonly called Heiss right angled forceps. Lahey's right angled forceps can be commonly confused with the curved angle forceps. These forceps called the Mixters forceps are curved but not to a right angle.

Langenbeck Retractor (Fig. 18.10)

The Langenbeck retractor is one of the most commonly used retractors in minor and superficial surgeries. This retractor has its blades at right angles to the instrument. It can be used to retract the soft tissue during surgery like hernia repair or appendectomy.The handle has a gap in between to make the instrument light weight. It resembles the "L" letter. A variant of the Langenbeck retractor is the **Richardson retractor** which has similar blades at both the ends.

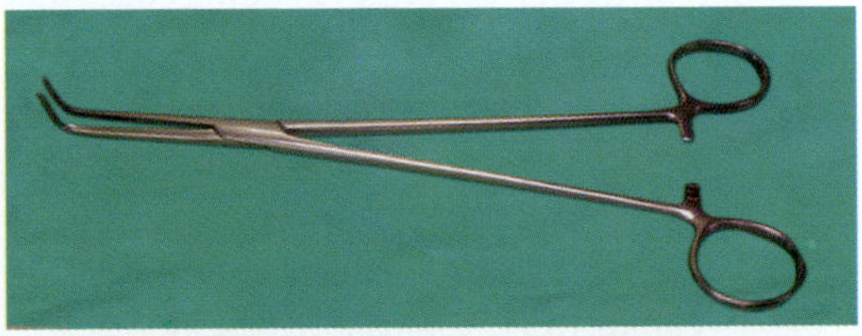

Figure 18.9: Lahey's right angled forceps

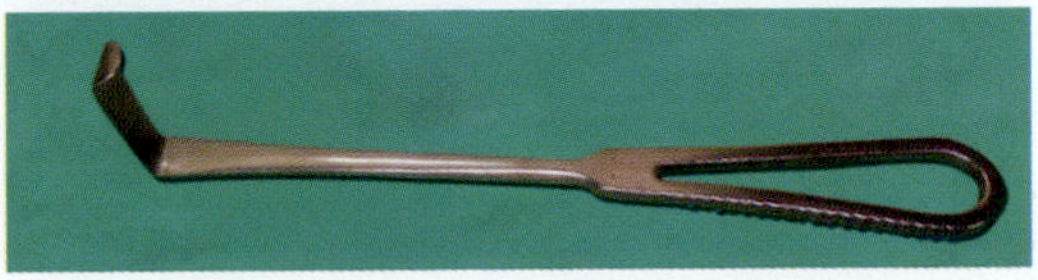

Figure 18.10: Langenbeck retractor

Volkmann's/Cat Paw/Rake Retractor (Fig. 18.11)

Volkmann's cat paw retractor is also used in superficial surgeries involving the skin and subcutaneous tissue. Some of its common applications are to retract soft tissue during venesection or excision biopsy The Volkmann's retractor has multiple small hooks at its end which retracts the superficial flap. One of its variant with a single hook is called Vicky's retractor. When the Rake retractor is combined with a Langenbeck blade at the other end it is commonly referred to as the Senn retractor.

Roberts Artery Forceps (Fig. 18.12)

Roberts artery forceps is a pair of long artery forceps useful for dissection and assisting in haemostasis in deeper regions of the abdomen. Some of its common uses are:

- Insertion of abdominal drains or intercostal drainage tubes
- Can be used to pass free ties especially in the pelvic surgery

Metzenbaum Dissection Scissors/ Tissue Cutting Scissors (Fig. 18.13)

Named after the American surgeon Myron Firth Metzenbaum, these scissors are used for cutting delicate soft tissue. They are different form the heavy Mayo Scissors in being lighter, slender and having a longer handle. Metzenbaum scissors may be coated with tungsten carbide cutting edges that provide a finer cut and are recognized by their gold-plated ring handles.

Kocher's Forceps (Fig. 18.14)

Named after Emil Kocher, a German born Swiss surgeon, Kocher's forceps are a type of toothed forceps with a long flat area to crush tissue in between. It is commonly used to:

- Hold tough fascia like the rectus sheath during laparotomy
- Artificial rupture of membrane
- May be used to crush the stump of appendix
- Hold the loop formed by umbilical tape or infant feeding tube during isolation of the spermatic cord, ureter.

Czerny's Retractor (Fig. 18.15)

It is a non-self-retaining retractor with a bi-flanged hook at one end and a blade at the other end, both perpendicular to the instrument. The centre is

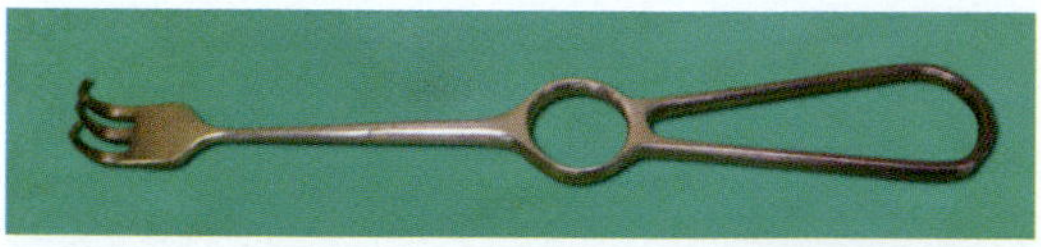

Figure 18.11: Volkmann's retractor

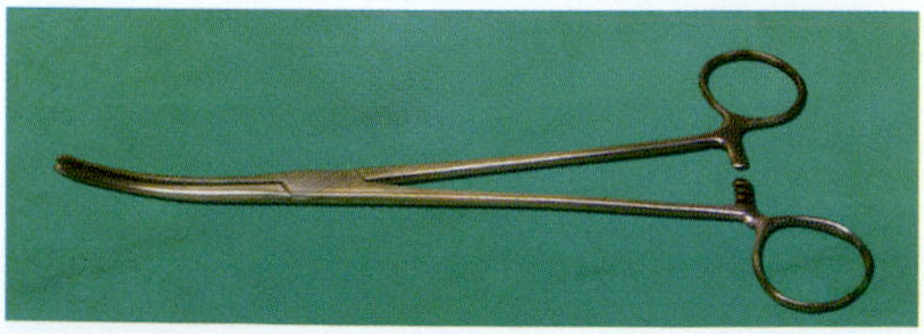

Figure 18.12: Roberts artery forceps

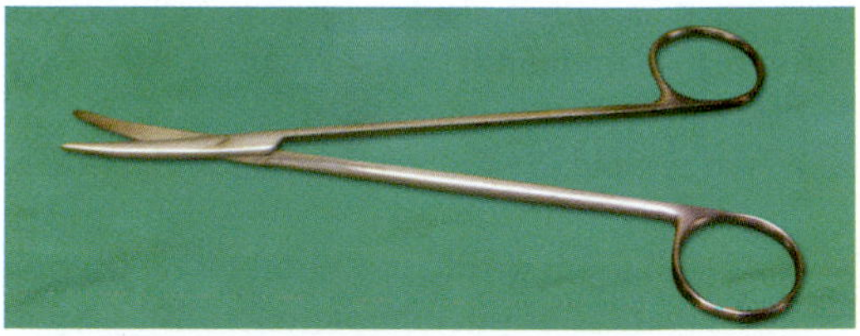

Figure 18.13: Metzenbaum dissection scissors

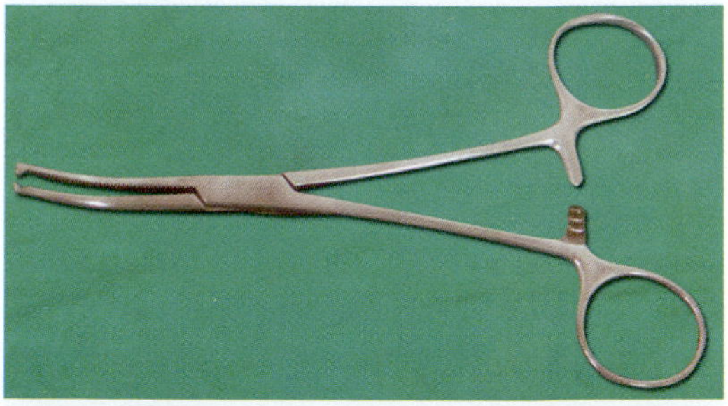

Figure 18.14: Kocher's forceps

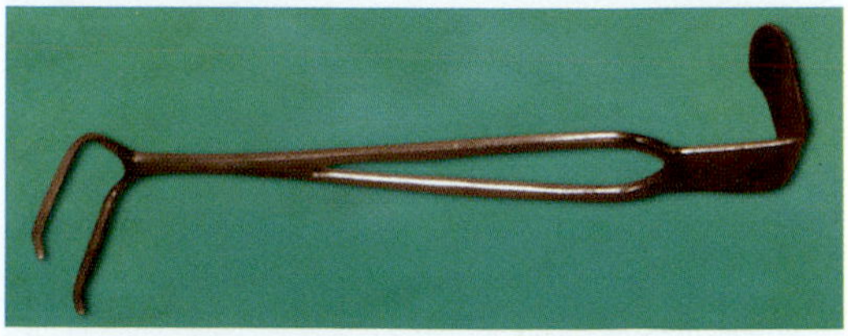

Figure 18.15: Czerny's retractor

fenestrated to make the instrument light weight. It has a bi-flanged hook at one end which can be used to retract the tail end of the wound, while sutures can be placed in the space between the two hooks. Czerny's retractor is used to retract the margins of the incision during laparotomy, appendicectomy and cholecystectomy. It is mainly used for superficial retraction. Its shape resembles the English alphabet "Z".

Desjardin's Forceps (Fig. 18.16)

Desjardin's forceps have a screw joint with the tip designed to firmly hold the stone. They do not have serrations but have a central fenestration which helps in the lodgement of the stone. Desjardin's forceps are used to extract stones from the common bile duct.

Randall's Stone Holding Forceps

Randall's stone holding forceps are very similar to the Desjardin's forceps in construction with the only differences being the serrations on the tips and the curved working ends. The Randall's forceps are available with working ends in various angles ranging from 60°–270°. These angles facilitate the approach and removal of stones from calyces which are placed at varied angles in relation to the pelvis. Serrations provide a better grip for these harder renal calculi.

Spencer Well's Haemostatic Forceps (Fig. 18.17)

These forceps are commonly used as a hemostat, or as a pedicle clamp and are perhaps the most versatile forceps available to the general surgeon. They can be employed for tissue holding, haemostasis, dissection and even holding a suture needle in the case of dire emergencies or when applying fine sutures. Spencer Well's forceps can also be used to drain an abscess cavity in the same fashion as a Hilton's abscess forceps but with greater care to avoid damage to the deeper structures. Due to their versatility they are available in various sizes ranging from very small (Mosquito/Halsted) to large (Kelly's).

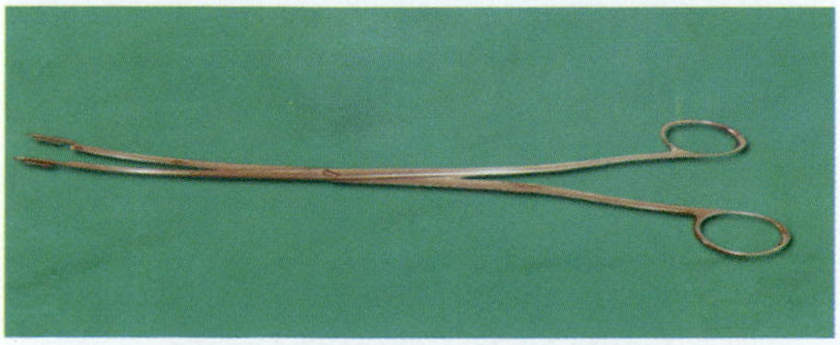

Figure 18.16: Desjardin's forceps

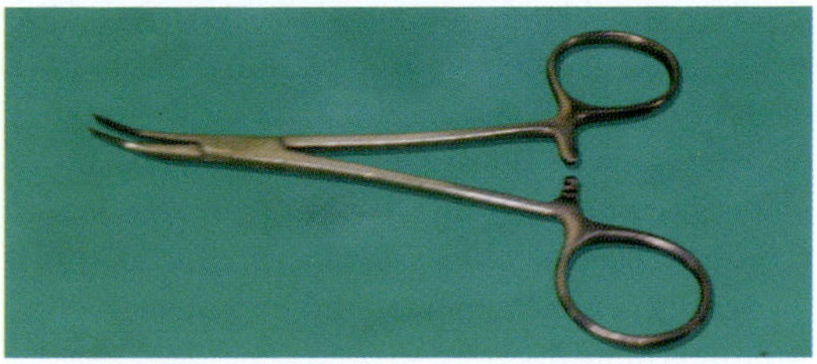

Figure 18.17: Spencer Well's haemostatic forceps

Tissue Dissection Forceps/Pickups/ Adson's Forceps (Fig. 18.18)

Tissue dissection forceps is used to hold delicate tissue for traction and counter traction during dissection. The Adson's forceps has some transverse serrations in the tips to provide a better hold but is non toothed. The toothed variants are also available and used to hold tough structures like the sheaths and thick fascia.

Bulldog's Vascular Clamp (Fig. 18.19)

The Bulldog's vascular clamp is a spring-loaded crossover clamp for vessels, to stop blood flow distal and proximal to the site of ongoing vascular repair. It is the most versatile clamp used in vascular surgery and has longitudinal striations

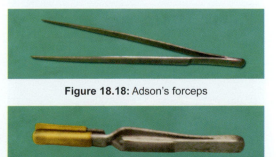

Figure 18.18: Adson's forceps

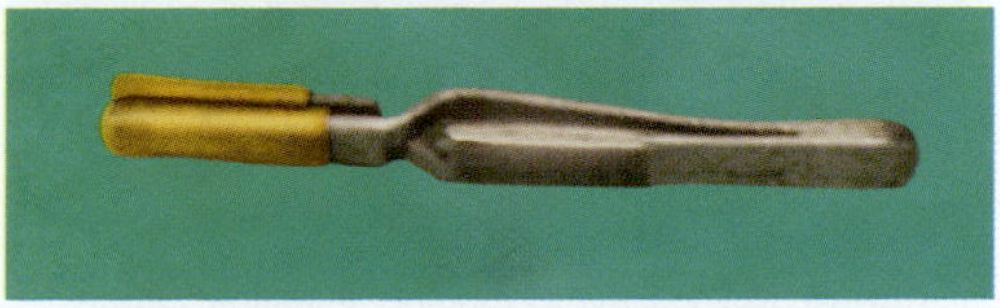

Figure 18.19: Bulldog's vascular clamp

along its tips like the deBakey's forceps and other vascular instruments. The working ends have been modified to suit all kinds of vessels and may be long, curved or straight. In the figure shown below the ends are covered with rubber shots to prevent damage to vessel wall. This is also how the instrument is usually stored to protect the fine striations at its tip.

Doyen's Intestinal Forceps/Non-crushing Intestinal Clamps (Fig. 18.20)

Doyen's intestinal forceps or clamps are used to temporarily occlude the lumen of the bowel. These clamps are designed to only occlude the lumen of the bowel without causing any physical damage to the wall of the gut. Compared to the crushing intestinal clamps which are more heavy duty and are apposed very tightly, space is appreciable between the two blades of the Doyen's clamp until the instrument is locked. The blades are light weight and fit snugly into each other. They have longitudinal serrations which cause minimal pressure necrosis and damage.

Payr's Crushing Intestinal/Pyloric Clamp (Fig. 18.21)

Payr's crushing clamps use a double lever mechanism to occlude and crush the bowel lumen while performing resection of gut. The instrument closes in two stages, the first lock wherein the bowel lumen is occluded and the second lock wherein the wall is crushed between the blades. To resect a part of the gut two crushing clamps are applied to the ends of the diseased gut and two noncrushing clamps applied 5 cm from the crushing clamp on both the ends on the healthy part of the gut. The gut is transected between the crushing and noncrushing clamp and the healthy gut is anastomosed to each other or brought out as a stoma. Another variant of the crushing intestinal clamp used in gastric resection is known as the Rochester-Pean clamp.

Allis Forceps (Fig. 18.22)

Allis forceps is a haemostatic forceps used to hold fibrous structures like the rectus sheath during laparotomy. It can also be used as a hemostat. The Allis forceps has splayed out tips with fine serrations which grip the tissue.

Babcock's Forceps (Fig. 18.23)

Babcock's forceps is designed to handle tubular structures like the appendix, the ureter, and the fallopian tubes. The working ends hold the tubular structures with minimal tension so that the intraluminal effects are minimal.

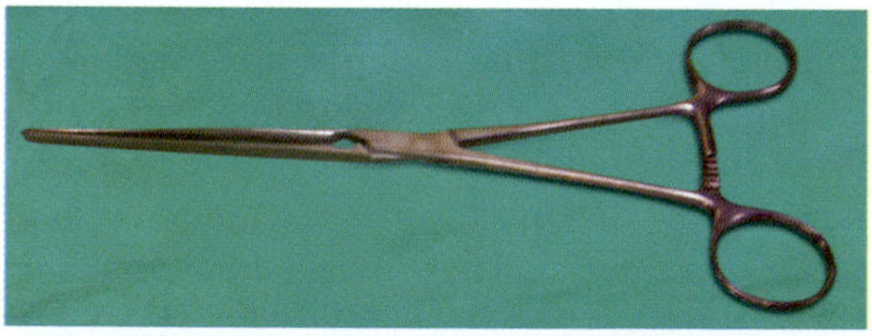

Figure 18.20: Doyen's intestinal clamp

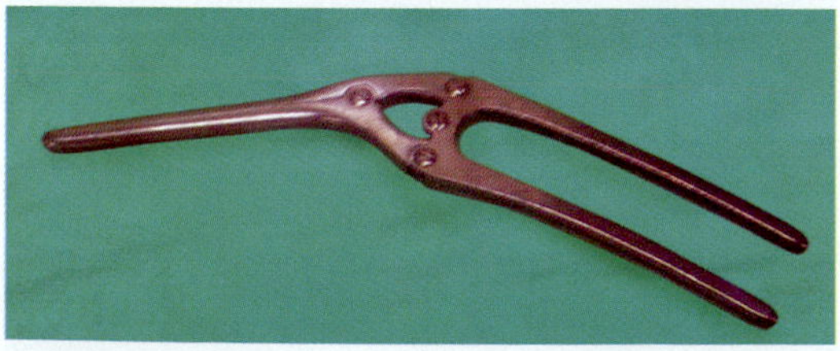

Figure 18.21: Payr's crushing intestinal clamp

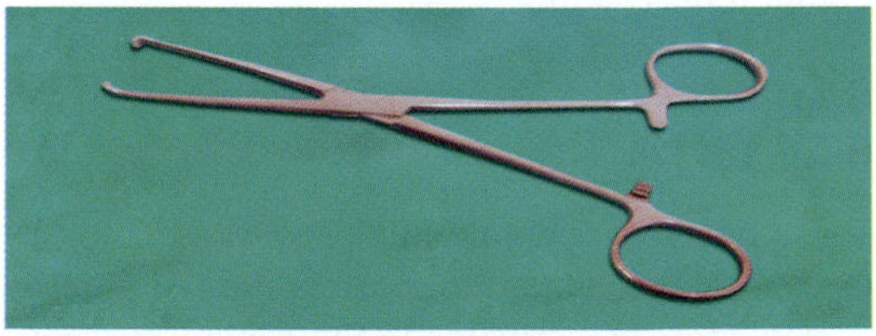

Figure 18.22: Allis forceps

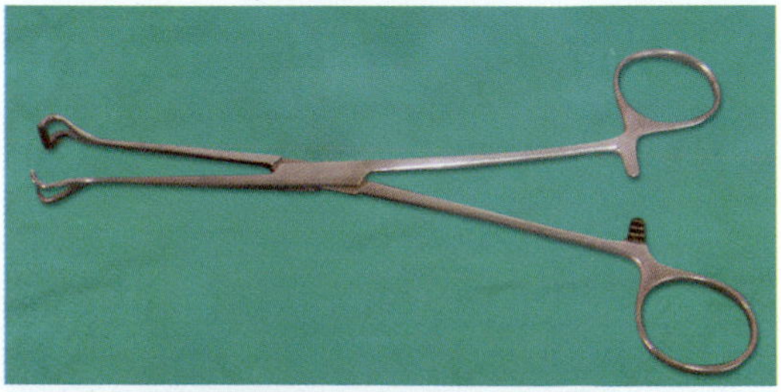

Figure 18.23: Babcock's forceps

BP Handle and Blades

The Bard Parker handle consists of a stainless steel handle with a mount on which a surgical blade is placed. Commonly used sizes are handle number 3 and 4. Blades of series 11–15 are mounted on the handle no 3, while blade number 20–30 which are larger blades are mounted on handle number 4. The mounted BP handle is grasped like a pen, and always transferred in a kidney dish.

Deaver's Retractor (Fig. 18.24)

Deaver's retractor is a single bladed curved retractor used to retract deep abdominal or chest incisions and viscera like the liver during cholecystectomy. It is available in various sizes and used widely in upper abdominal surgeries. A wet mop may be used as an interface when applying it to solid viscera like the liver or the spleen.

Morris Retractor (Fig. 18.25)

The Morris retractor is used to retract wound edges during abdominal operations. It has a blade at both ends which can snugly fit over the wound edge. Morris retractor is widely employed in laparotomy, pelvic surgeries and gynaecological surgeries.

Joll's Thyroid Retractor (Fig. 18.26)

Joll's thyroid retractor is a screw adjustable retractor bearing two spring action clips on its ends. Its width can be actively adjusted by a central roll over screw mechanism. The spring action clips have a release button at their lateral margins to demount the apparatus. This retractor is widely used in thyroid surgeries and other neck surgeries. Other commonly employed retractors for thyroid and neck surgery are the green goitre retractor and the Weitlaner retractor.

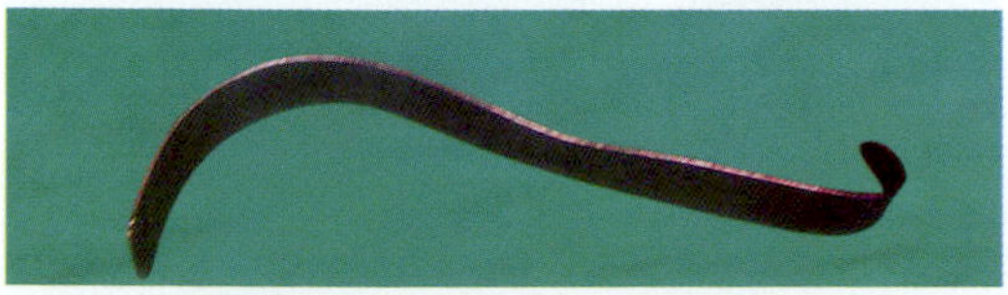

Figure 18.24: Deaver's retractor

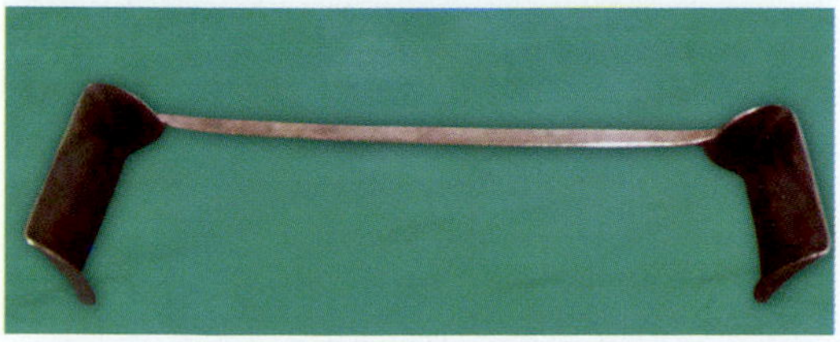

Figure 18.25: Morris retractor

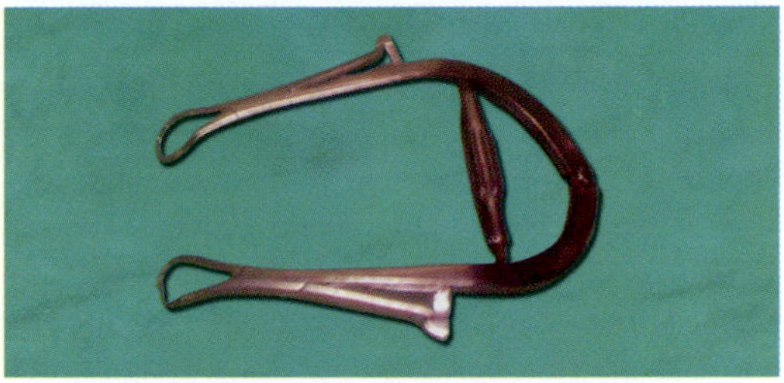

Figure 18.26: Joll's thyroid retractor

Balfour Self-retaining Abdominal Wall Retractor (Fig. 18.27)

Balfour abdominal retractor places blades over a pair of channels with a lock, of which one is fixed and the other one can be slided over the channel and retained in its position. This instrument is used in laparotomies and lower abdominal surgeries. It eliminates the use of active traction by the assistant.

DeBakey's Vascular Forceps

DeBakey's forceps belong to the DeBakey's series of instruments with characteristic longitudinal serrations. The serrations are small with two longitudinal grooves which hold the vessel without crushing. Vessels are best held by the adventitia to cause minimal damage to endothelium.

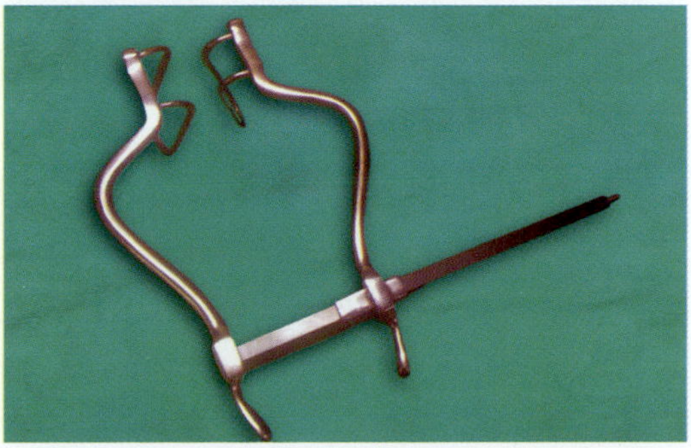

Figure 18.27: Balfour self-retaining abdominal wall retractor

Cooley Satinsky Clamp (Fig. 18.28)

Named after Dr Victor P Satinsky, the Cooley Satinsky clamp is used to clamp the vessel during repair or perform vascular end to side or side-to-side anastomosis. The section to be repaired is placed in the concavity of the clamp and the distal and proximal flow is occluded by locking the clamp. The working ends have longitudinal serrations to gently occlude the lumen.

Rampley's Sponge Holding Forceps (Fig. 18.29)

Rampley's sponge holding forceps has ringed tips with transverse serrations that provide a good grip for holding objects. It is commonly used for:

- Swabbing the operative field for disinfection
- Holding the sponge and swabbing the vagina
- Applying medication to deep seated areas
- Applying pressure over the small areas which are oozing
- Grasping the gallbladder during open cholecystectomy.

Lister/Bandage Scissors

Lister's or bandage cutting scissors have a broad blade on one side and a normal second blade. One of its variant used to cut plaster or thick dressings has a blunt tip in front of one of its blades which is broader than the second blade. These scissors are heavier and the blunt tip prevents accidental injury to the body when the blade is introduced between the skin and the dressing.

Cheek Retractor (Fig. 18.30)

Cheek retractors are available in a variety of designs, being self-retracting as well as non-self-retracting. These retractors are useful in surgeries on the cheek, oral cavity, tongue and the maxilla. The blades of the cheek retractor fit in the vestibular area between the lips and the gums and the self-retaining mechanism, usually in the form of a spring keeps the oral cavity wide open. The classical single piece non-self-retaining cheek retractor is also applied in a similar fashion and traction is applied laterally by the assistant.

Thomson Walker's Cystolithotomy Forceps (Fig. 18.31)

The cystolithotomy forceps are designed with a cup-shaped working end with multiple spikes in the concavity to firmly grip the stone during open cystolithotomy. One of the rings is open and the other ring is complete.

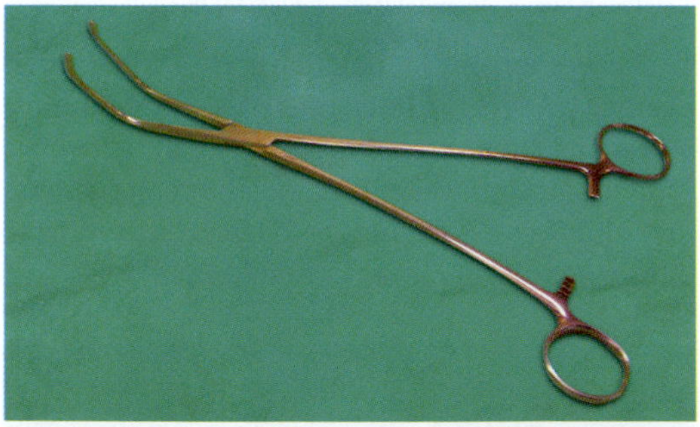

Figure 18.28: Satinsky clamp

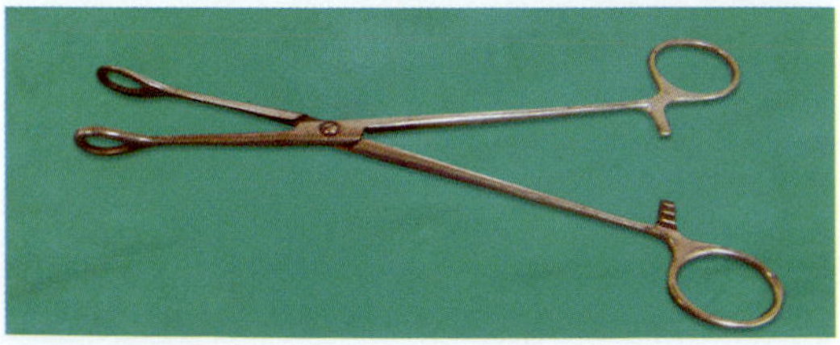

Figure 18.29: Sponge holding forceps

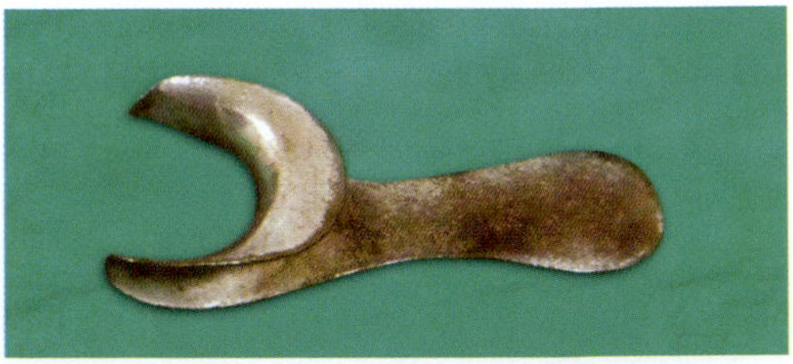

Figure 18.30: Cheek retractor

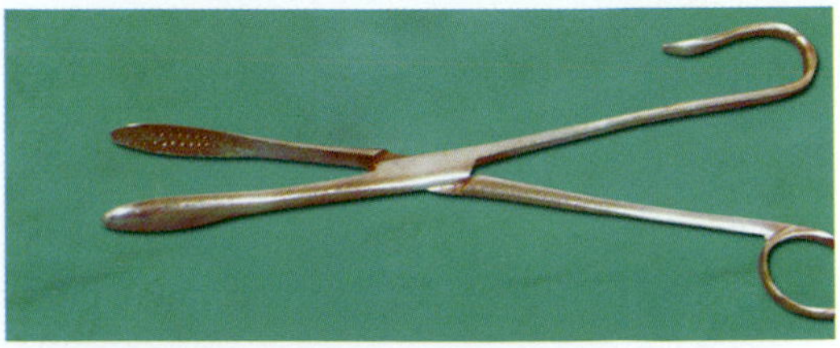

Figure 18.31: Thomson Walker's cystolithotomy forceps

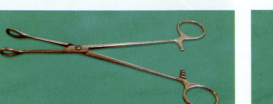

Alexander Farabeuf's Periosteal Elevator (Fig. 18.32)

Farabeuf's periosteal elevator is used to elevate the periosteum from the underlying bone. It has a sharp edge which peels off the periosteum along with attached muscles and ligaments from the bone. The edged end is connected to a shaft with a grip. It is commonly used in renal surgeries where the ligaments and muscles are shaved off the ribs during the flank approach.

Doyen Rib Raspatory (Fig. 18.33)

Rib raspatory is used to denude the rib of all the musculoaponeurotic attachments. It consists of a tubular shaft coiling and tapering at its end into a sharp marginated blade and a handle to which the shaft is attached. The raspatory is designed differently for use on the right or the left side. For identification the raspatory is placed on the level surface and the side to which the coil is open is the side where it is applied from the inferior edge onwards encircling the whole rib devoiding it of its periosteum.

Rib Cutter (Fig. 18.34)

The rib cutter is used to cut off the rib after it has been cleared of all the attachments. If there is continuous bleed from the bone ends after cutting the rib, bone wax may be applied to the fresh end.

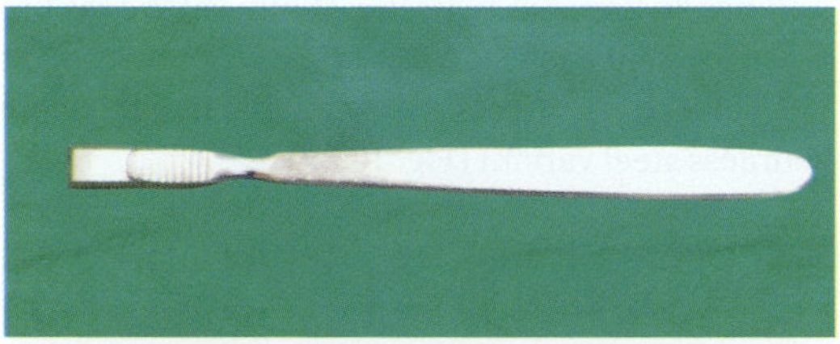

Figure 18.32: Periosteal elevator

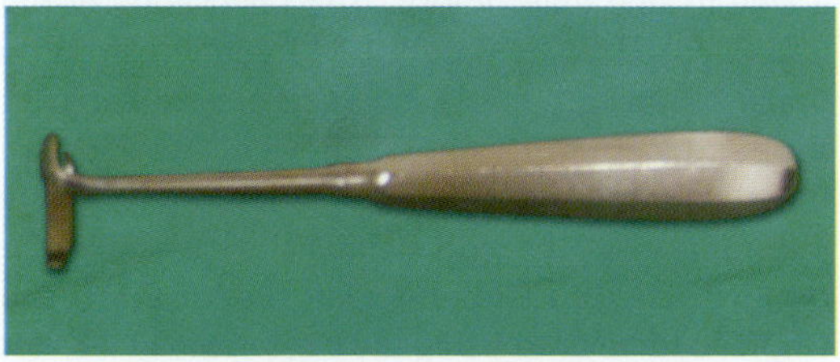

Figure 18.33: Rib raspatory

Rib is cut during the flank approach if the exposure of the kidney is compromised.

Finochietto Chest Wall Retractor (Fig. 18.35)

Unlike the abdominal wall which is flexible, the thoracic wall is much less pliable and requires much stronger retraction. This is possible with the Finochietto chest wall retractor which is a self-retaining retractor with two blades and a rack and pinion arrangement to retract them as required. Being a strong mechanical device it is important to prevent damage to delicate viscera.

Nerve Hook (Fig. 18.36)

This is used to hook and raise nerve during various procedures, e.g. lumbar sympathectomy, transposition of ulnar nerve. This helps in dissection of nerve.

Vein Hook (Fig. 18.37)

This instrument is useful in dissecting and lifting the veins during avulsion of perforators or localised dilated veins.

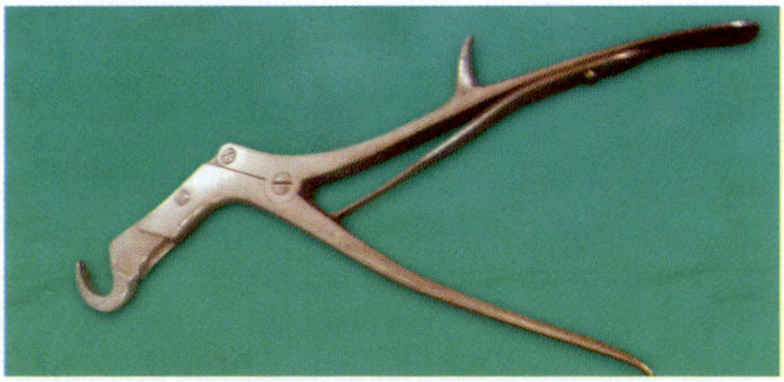

Figure 18.34: Rib cutter

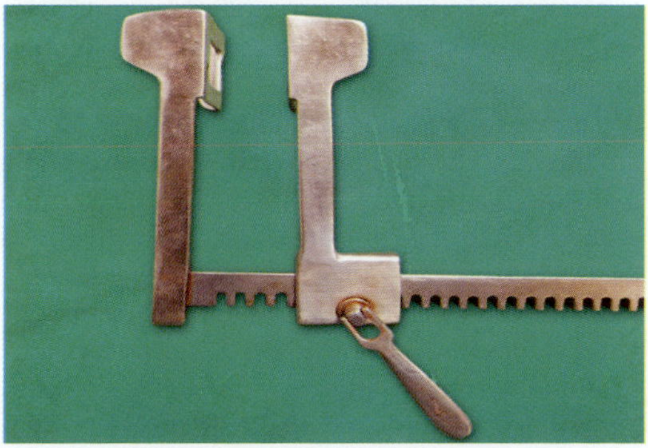

Figure 18.35: Chest wall retractor

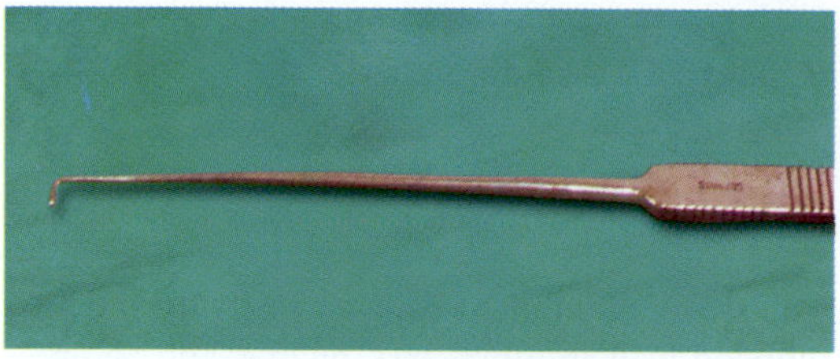

Figure 18.36: Nerve hook

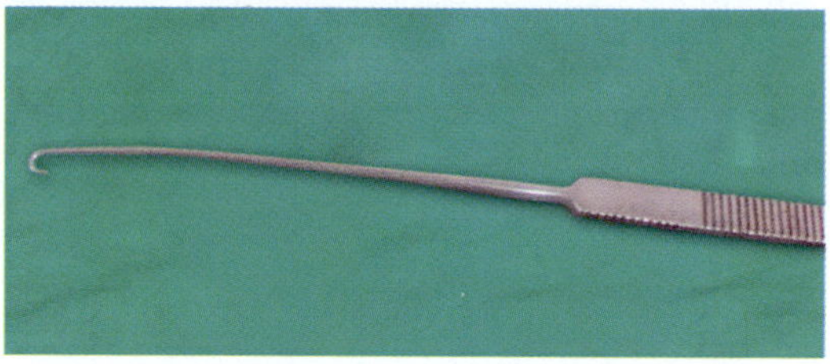

Figure 18.37: Vein hook

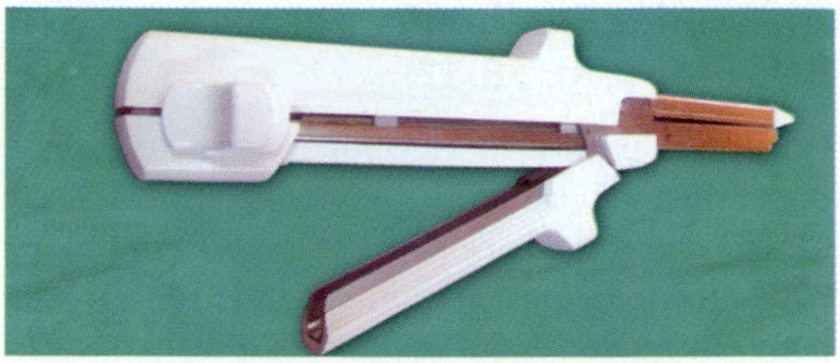

Figure 18.38: Linear cutter

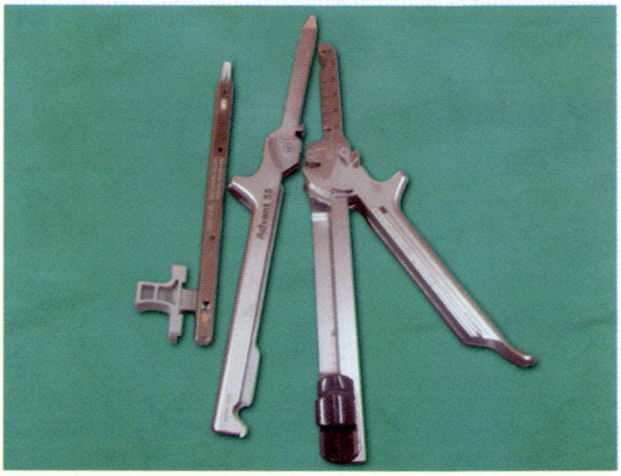

Figure 18.39: Reusable stainless steel variant of the linear cutter

SECTION 2: STAPLERS

Staplers and their applications in surgery have already been discussed in the earlier sections of this book. In this section the commonly used stapling devices have been arranged, to induce familiarity with these new advancements in the field of surgery.

Disposable Linear Cutter (Fig. 18.38)

The disposable linear cutter has two halves and a cartridge. The two halves are engaged into each other and the cartridge is loaded between the two blades. The various cartridges have colour codes which determine the depth to which the stapler can penetrate. The vascular structures can be anastomosed using the grey and white cartridges, while thicker structures like the intestine require the blue or green cartridge. Once engaged over the tissue to be divided, the instrument is locked and fired by closing the bar on the right side of the instrument and cut by sliding the handle over the groove. While engaging the stapler on the tissue to be divided, the slider must always face the surgeon. The slider is dealt with the thenar aspect of the hand. Once the stapler is fired, some surgeons would advocate a waiting period of 30 seconds to achieve haemostasis before the tissue is cut. After the completion of the division the tissue cavity must be inspected for any active bleeding which can be dealt with active compression by a gauze or over running sutures. The linear cutter can be used for performing side-to-side anastomosis.

These linear cutters with blue or green cartridges fires two rows of staples on each side and divide tissue in between. White cartridges fire three rows on each side.

The linear cutter is also available in a reusable stainless steel variant (Fig. 18.39).

Transverse Intestinal Stapler (TIA) (Fig. 18.40)

Transverse stapler is also employed while fashioning a side-to-side anastomosis. The open ends of the anastomosed tissue (Performed initially using the linear cutter) are engaged in the groove between the two parts of this stapling device. The ends are initially approximated using the knob with screw like motion at the end of this device. Once the tissue is engaged and uniformly fits the grove, the stapler can be fired using the trigger. Since it is not a cutter, the tissue remaining above the staple line

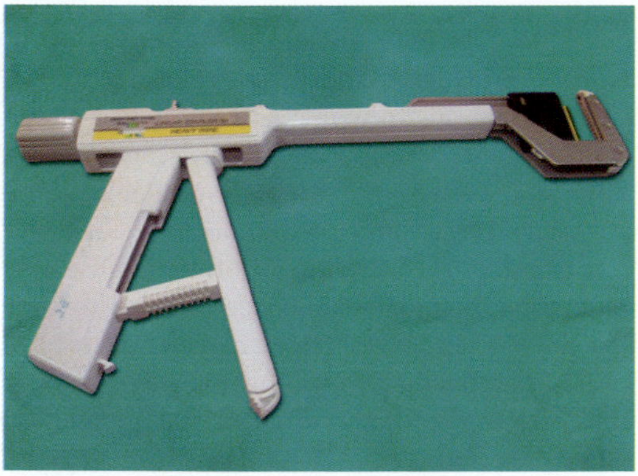

Figure 18.40: TIA stapler

can be cut by running a scalpel in the stainless steel groove provided in the instrument. The TIA are also available in various sizes depending upon the length of anastomosis and the type of gut utilised.

Circular Stapler (Fig. 18.41)

The circular stapler is devised to perform the end-to-end anastomosis. It has two essential components the anvil and the stapling device. The anvil is first engaged in the proximal part of gut, and purse string sutures applied to secure it in the lumen. The distal part of the device is introduced through the distal gut or the anal canal lumen of which is already occluded in the proximal aspect. The sharp end of the anvil pierces the occluded end of the distal gut and engages into the stapler. Once the device is engaged the screw knob at the distal end of the device is turned to bring the two ends in the firing safe zone which is indicated by a coloured indicator incorporated in the handle of this device. When the indicator turns green, indicating that the anastomosis is safe to perform, the stapling device is fired by using the trigger. The anastomosis is performed along with cutting of the excess gut tissue in the form of a doughnut which is checked for adequacy and complete circumference once the device is disengaged. As with other types of stapling devices the haemostasis and adequacy of anastomosis are essentially confirmed intraoperatively.

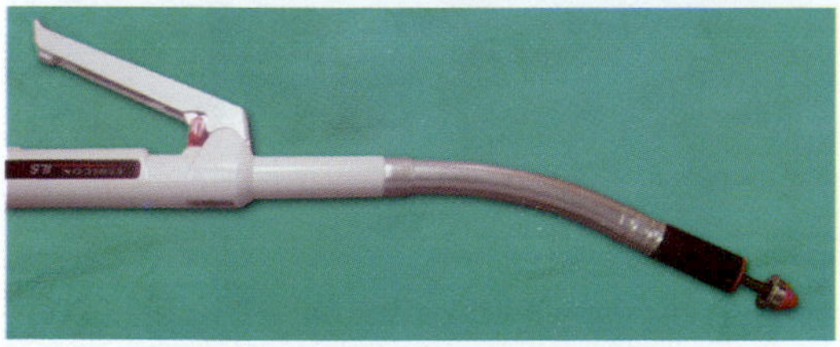

Figure 18.41: Circular stapler

Laparoscopic Linear Stapler (Fig. 18.42)

Introduced through a 12 mm port, this device functions in essentially the same way as the linear cutter. It has two triggers, one to engage the stapler and the other to cut the tissue. It is a disposable and costly device available in various sizes and cartridge lengths.

Laparoscopic Transverse Stapler (Fig. 18.43)

This is the laparoscopic variant of the TIA, which has the same construction as the laparoscopic linear stapler with two triggers and an additional flexible head to engage the open ends for transverse stapling.

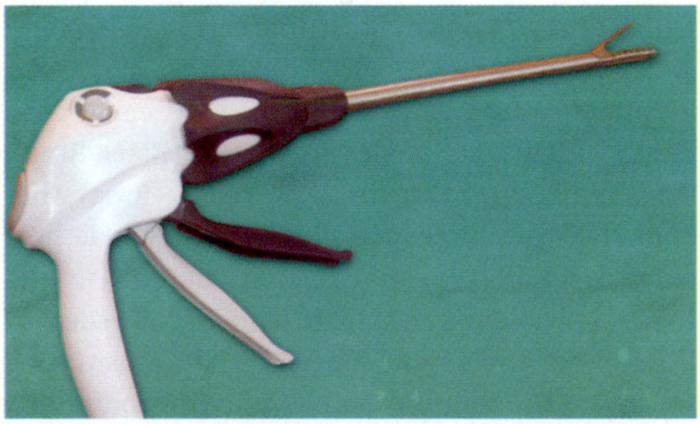

Figure 18. 42: Laparoscopic linear stapler

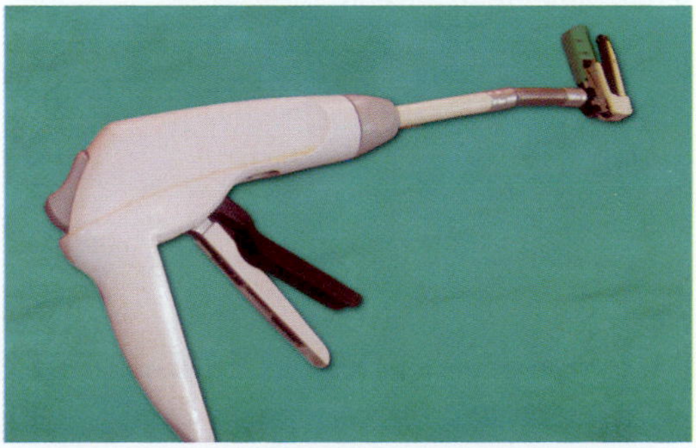

Figure 18.43: Laparoscopic transverse stapler

BASIC LAPAROSCOPIC INSTRUMENTS

The Verees Needle (Fig. 18.44)

The Verees needle is a specially designed needle used for creating pneumoperitoneum by the closed method. This needle was devised by Janos Verees in 1932 and consists of a spring loaded stylet in a 14 gauge needle which is about 15 cm long. The blunt tip recedes back exposing the sharp outer sheath when it encounters resistance. On hitting soft tissue such as the viscera, it is the blunt needle that is encountered, thereby protecting these tissues from penetrating injury. The needle has high flow stopcock which can allow gas flow up to 2.5 litres/min.

The Laparoscope

The laparoscope consists of a Hopkins Rod Lens system with intervening vacuum encased in a stainless steel tube. Around this system is a series of fibre optic cables that transmit light from the light source. The Laparoscope can be a straight viewing one which is also called a 0° scope and identified by a green ring on the light cable port. Other widely used angles are the 12° (Black Ring), 30° (Red Ring), and the 70° (Yellow Ring). The angled scopes are especially useful in single port surgeries and are an effective solution to the rollover problems. The laparoscope is connected to the camera and a fibre optic cable for transmitting images to the monitor and light to the abdominal cavity. The new generation laparoscopes feature a flexible tip and a CCD camera at the tip of the scope rather than the end.

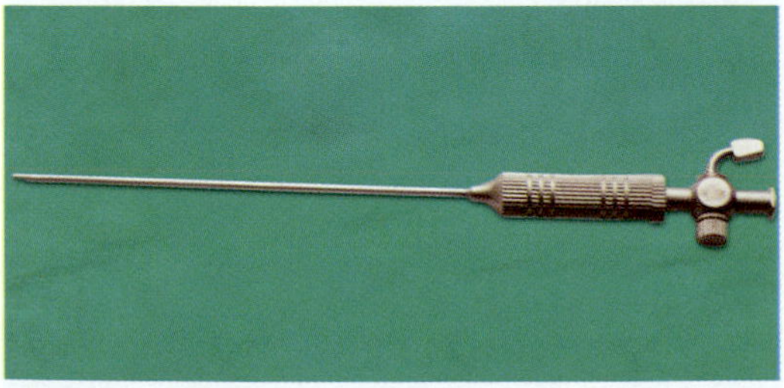

Figure 18.44: Verees needle

Trocars (Fig. 18.45)

Trocars provide a sheath for introduction of laparoscopic instruments and minimise tissue damage and complications in laparoscopic surgery. A variety of trocars are available to the minimal access surgeon and include the solid core pointed trocars, bladed trocars and the new generation nonbladed and see-through trocars. The shielded and nonshielded bladed trocars have largely been replaced by the bladeless trocars. These trocars are made up of plastic and can be safely inserted using a corkscrew movement. Apart from minimising the risk of injury to bowel or vessels these trocars obviate the need of fascial closure of port sites. The see-through ports (visual obturator port) allow the operator to see the abdominal wall layers as the port passes through them making them an excellent option of establishing pneumoperitoneum by the open method. Once the trocar is inserted, it can be connected to the gas inflow.

Light Source (Fig. 18.46)

Light is generated by a high power light bulb. This can be a white light source like xenon or incandescent light from a Halogen lamp. Light is made to pass through special filters and its temperature is reduced as it exits the light source unit. By means of fibreoptic cables the light reaches the laparoscope and illuminates the working space.

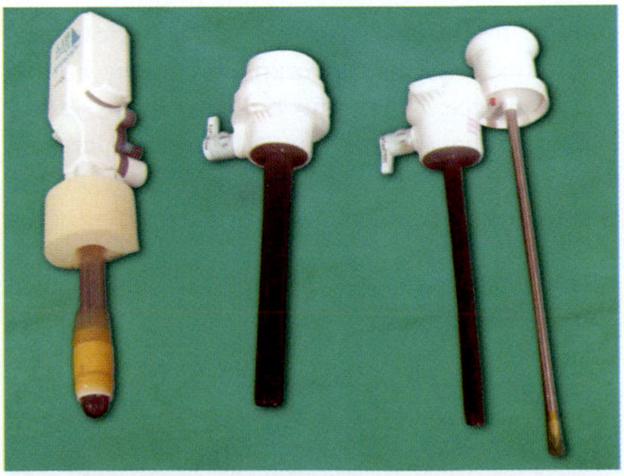

Figure 18.45: Various types of laparoscopic trocars

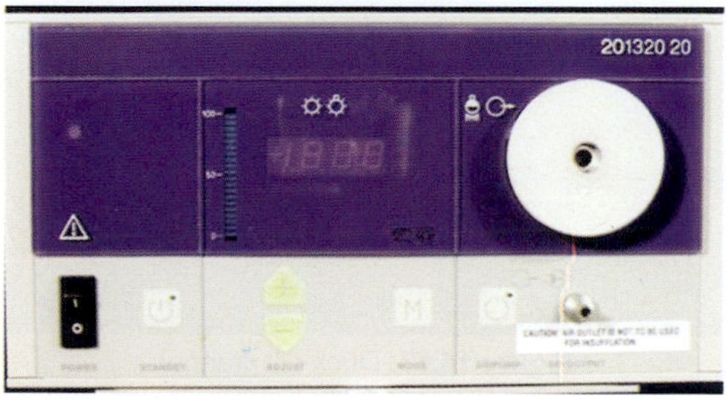

Figure 18.46: Light source

Insufflation Unit (Fig. 18.47)

The insufflation unit is responsible for inflation of gas in the peritoneal cavity, maintenance of intraperitoneal pressure at a desired value and a feedback loop to constantly monitor the abdominal pressure. The insufflation unit is connected to a gas cylinder.

Suction and Irrigation Unit (Fig. 18.48)

The suction irrigation unit connects a suction irrigation cannula to a suction bottle and a sterile saline solution which can be used for suction and irrigation respectively, at the touch of a button placed on the cannula. The irrigation fluid can be delivered at specified flow rates and suction done at low, medium or high pressures.

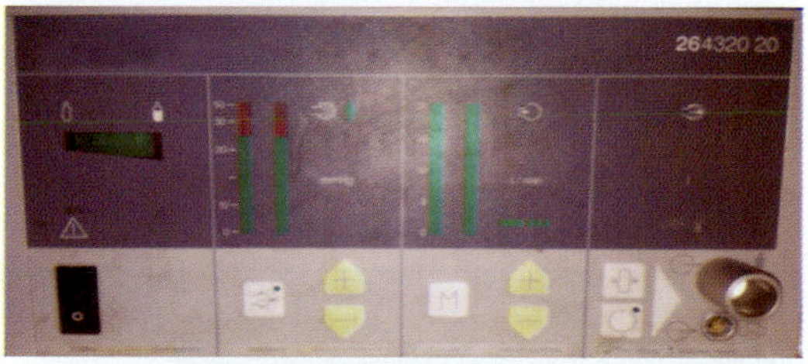

Figure 18.47: Insufflation unit

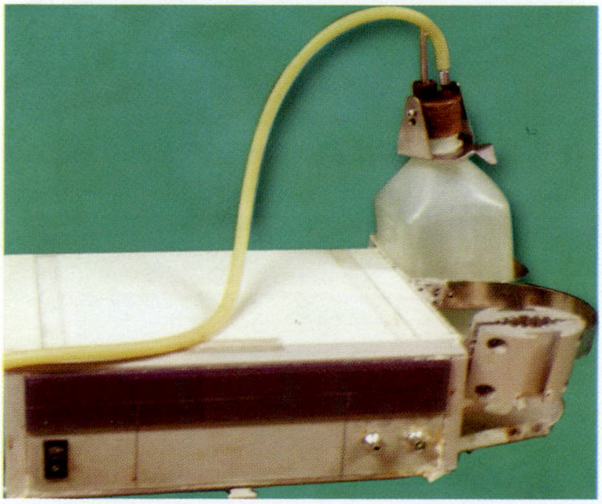

Figure 18.48: Suction and irrigation unit

Overview of Various Laparoscopic Surgery Instruments (Figs 18.49 to 18.63)

The gamut of laparoscopic instruments today is essentially a modification of the contemporary open surgical instruments. The handle may be ratcheted or nonratcheted with a toggle switch to lock the jaws as needed. These instruments are 20–35 cm long with their fulcrum at the mid-point. Bariatric instruments may be up to 45 cm long.

Rat Tooth Grasping Forceps (Figs 18.49 and 18.50)

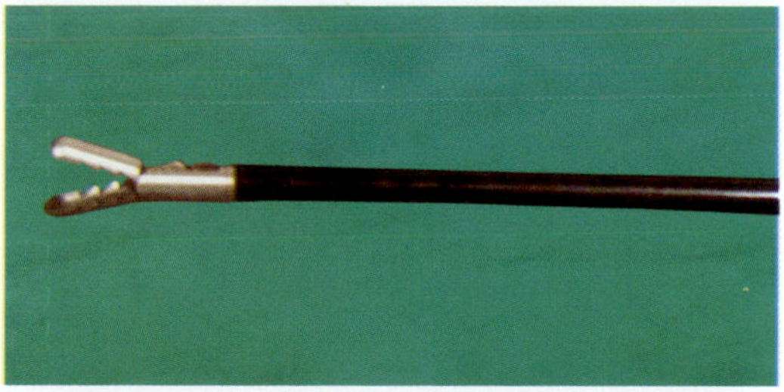

Figure 18.49: Short rat tooth grasping forceps

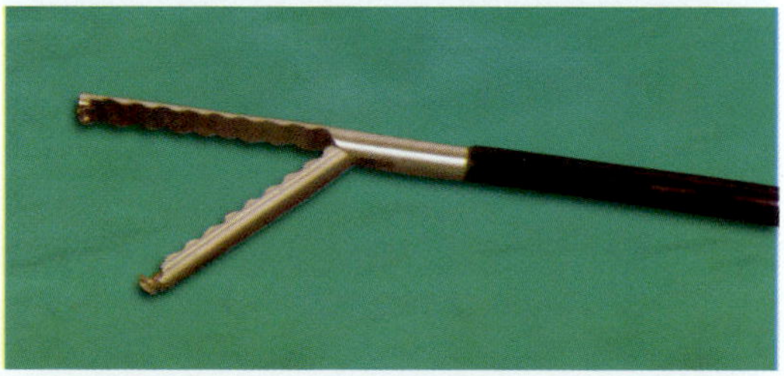

Figure 18.50: Long rat tooth grasping forceps

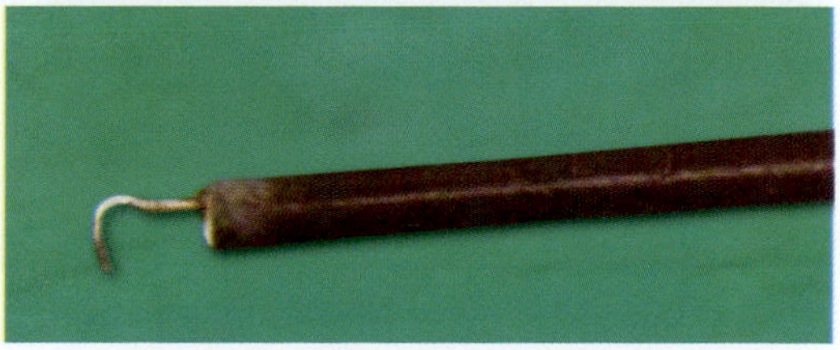

Figure 18.51: Electrosurgical hook

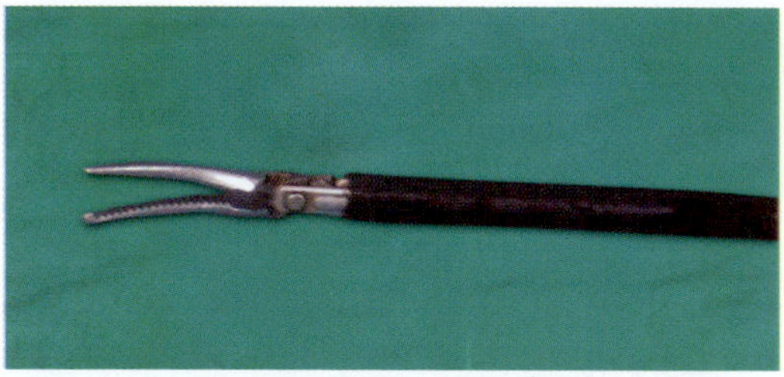

Figure 18.52: Maryland's dissector

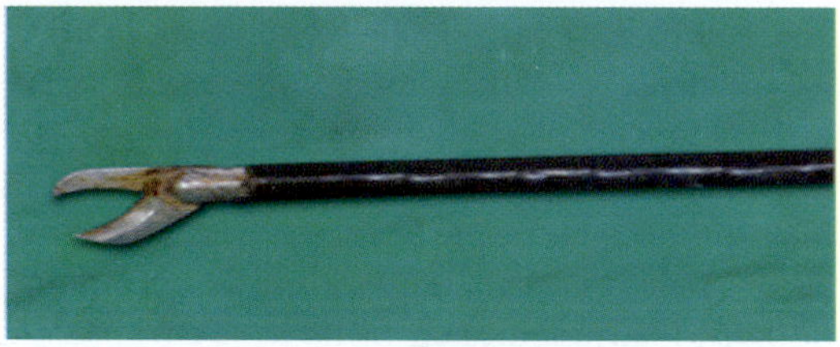

Figure 18.53: Hook scissors

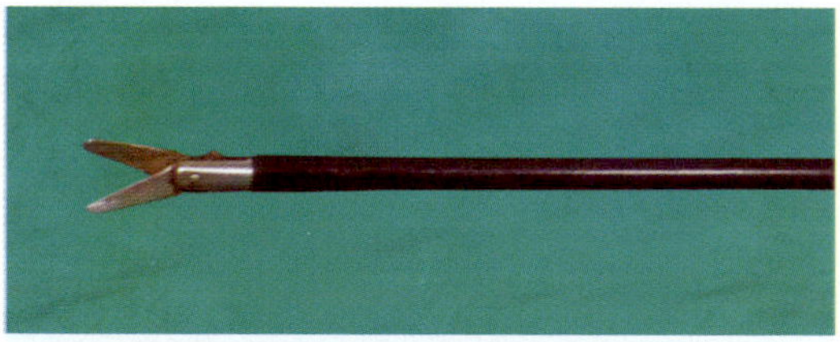

Figure 18.54: Metzenbaum scissors

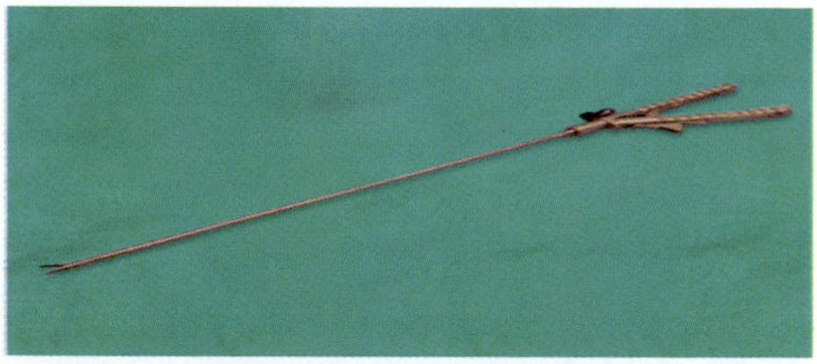

Figure 18.55: Needle holder

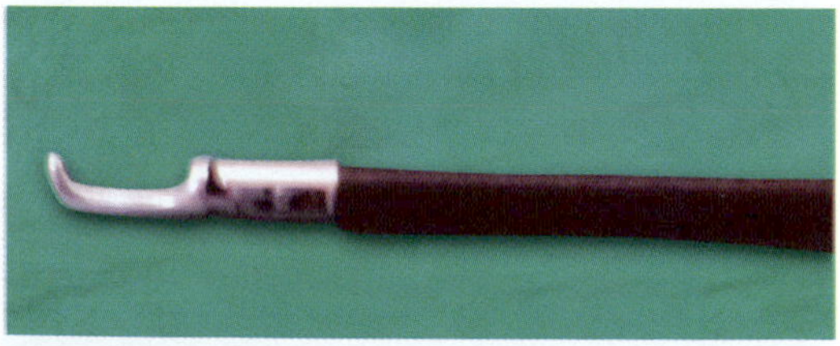

Figure 18.56: Crile dissection forceps

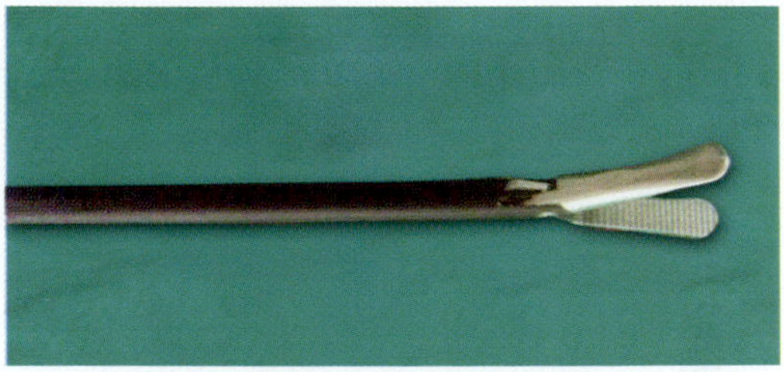

Figure 18.57: Duck bill grasper

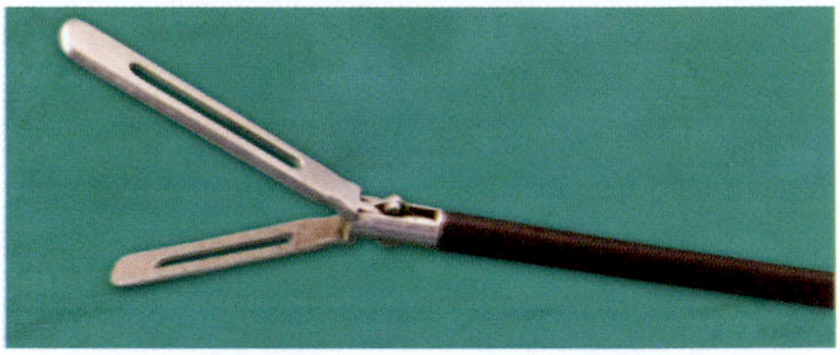

Figure 18.58: Dorsey intestinal forceps

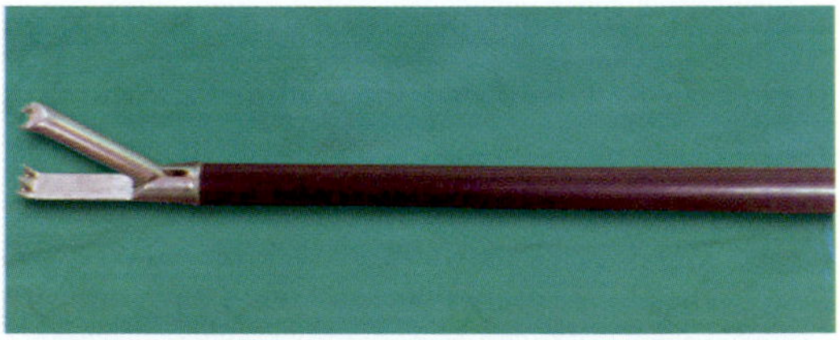

Figure 18.59: Claw grasper

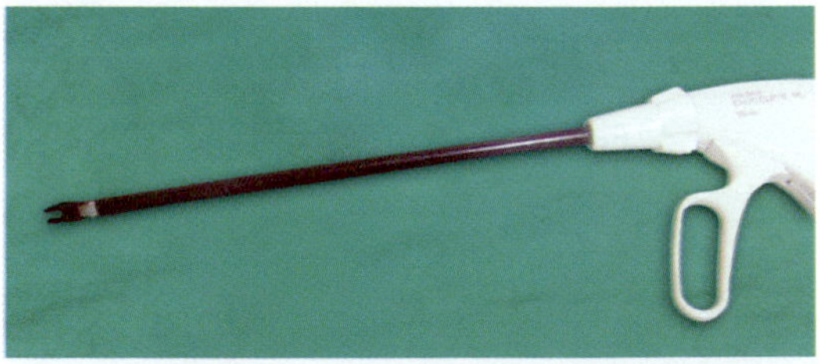

Figure 18.60: Clip applicator (Disposable)

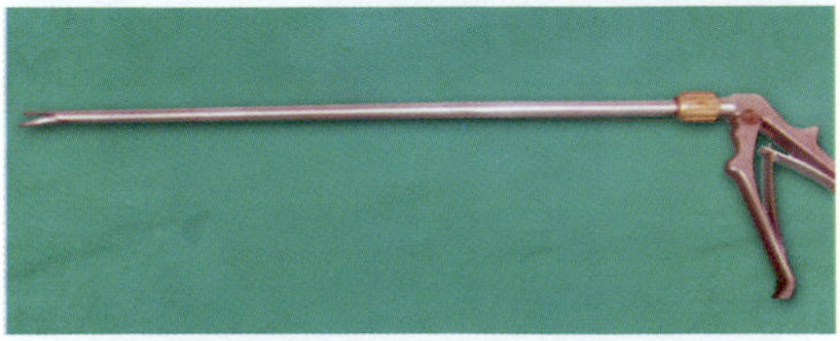

Figure 18.61A: Reusable clip applicator

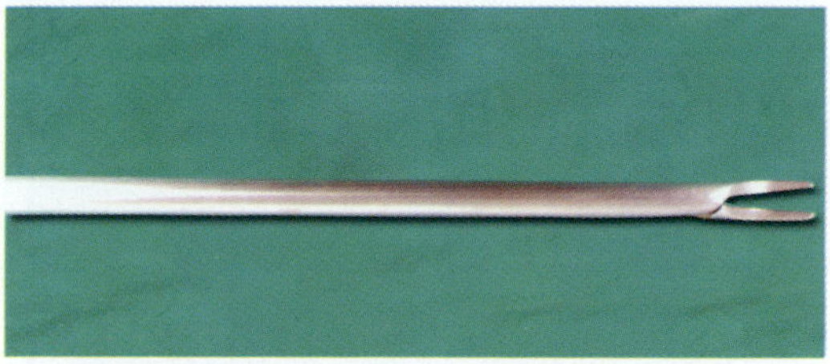

Figure 18.61B: Reusable clip applicator tip

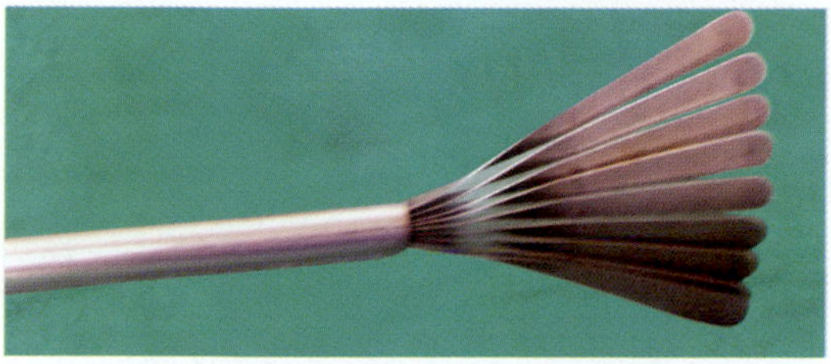

Figure 18.62: Fan-shaped retractor

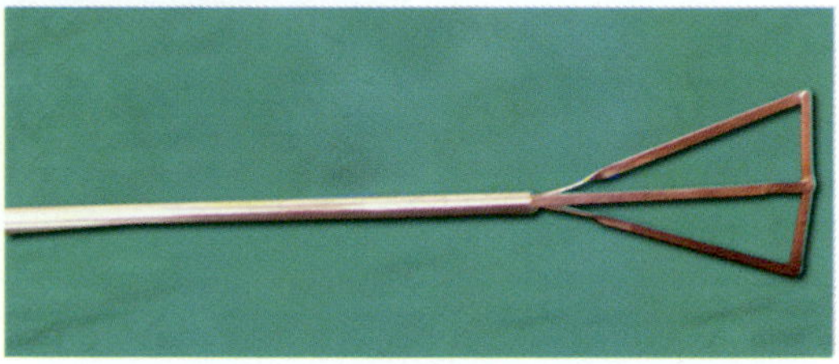

Figure 18.63: Trifflange retractor to retract liver, intestine, etc

Recent Developments of Energy Sources in Surgery

19

Raman Tanwar, Sudhir Kumar Jain

The field of surgery has seen a vast expansion with the amalgamation of technical advances with surgical principles. Energy in its various forms has been controlled and selectively applied in facilitating and minimising surgical trauma. Aim of this chapter is to outline the principles of various devices which use energy sources. These forms of energy include:

- Electric current is used in:
  a. Conventional monopolar and bipolar electrodes
  b. Feedback equipped bipolar systems, e.g. Ligasure®
  c. Radiofrequency ablation
- Ultrasonic waves: Ultrasonic dissector
- Electromagnetic waves: Used as microwaves, radiosurgery
- Cryoablation
- Light energy: Lasers, argon beam coagulation, photodynamic therapy, infrared coagulation
- With the advances in minimally invasive surgery, these sources are commonly used and aim of this chapter is outline the basic principles of these energy sources.

APPLICATION OF ELECTRIC CURRENT

The basic principles of application of electric current for haemostasis have already been covered previously in the chapter of electrocautery. With the advent of technological advances like incorporated impedance monitoring and feedback regulation of current it is possible to perform safer and reliable coagulation of tissue with minimal damage to surrounding tissue as the spread of current is minimal due to impedance monitoring. The commonly used devices employing these principles are Enseal®, PKS® and Ligasure® (Fig. 19.1). They are basically bipolar low voltage high current electrocautery devices which when activated after grasping the tissue send electrical current in a computer controlled fashion followed rapidly by a cycle of sensing tissue impedance and temperature at the site of action. Such cycles of monitoring the process of coagulation and providing appropriate energy in the next cycle takes place hundreds or thousands of times depending upon the device specification. These devices give audible signals to inform the operator of completion of the process of coagulation. The use of offset electrodes prevents lateral spread of current and minimises thermal damage to surrounding tissues.

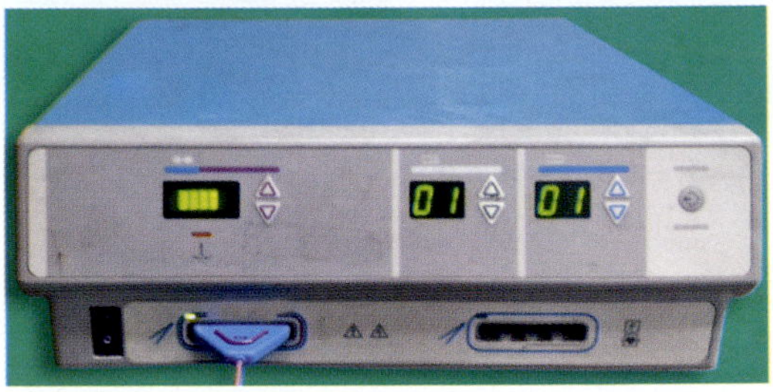

Figure 19.1: Ligasure generator is a type of bipolar impedance monitoring device

Mechanism of Action

These bipolar impedance devices act by a combination of bipolar current and pressure. A uniform pressure is applied to the tissues held between the soft jaws of the applicator to coagulate them. The applicator is connected to the generator which senses the various tissue impedance variables and decides the amount of energy that needs to be delivered in the next cycle. The device can be hand or foot activated.

There is denaturation of proteins and coaptation of vessels which makes these devices excellent tools to seal vessels. They provide bloodless dissection and can effectively seal vessels of diameters as large as 7 mm. These devices are superior over the conventional electrocautery. Cost of these devices limits its widespread use and application. Use of these devices saves time as surgeon does not have to tie vessels up to 7 mm.

RADIOFREQUENCY ABLATION

Radiofrequency ablation is a method for inducing tissue necrosis by using high frequency alternating current ranging from 350–500 kHz. Alternating in this frequency generates ionic agitation and cellular friction producing temperatures in the order of 80–100°C causing coagulative necrosis. The application can be controlled to generate areas of coagulation necrosis as large as 3–5 cm. Device works on the principle that when temperatures generated above 50°C is sustained for more than 3 minutes, it leads to denaturation of intracellular proteins along with loss of the bilayered lipid membrane leading to tissue death. This technology has been widely utilised for benign and malignant tumours and ablation of veins, nerves and cardiac tissue. The principle for all these applications remains the same with the types of probes varying according to the site of application. Radiofrequency ablation bears the advantage of being combined with other modalities of treatment and being used more than once to treat a lesion. It can be used percutaneously, laparoscopically as well as by open surgical approach. Percutaneous management of liver and renal tumours under image guidance is being extensively used to realise the potential and limitations of radiofrequency ablation.

Radiofrequency ablation can be applied to the conscious patient with morbidity approaching that of a tissue biopsy. Radiofrequency ablation is limited in application by the problems of charring of tissue and limited area of damage especially when applied close to a large vessel and therefore increased risk of residual disease. Addressing these issues manufacturers have come out with various design modifications and employment of cooling tip to reduce the charring and burning of tissue from heat. Impedance feedback can be added to the probes to provide more adequate tissue destruction.When the impedance rises rapidly the flow of current is cut off preventing further charring.

ULTRASONIC SHEARS (FIGS 19.2 AND 19.3)

Ultrasonic shears are a safer multipurpose instrument which can perform multiple tasks minimising instrument change with minimal lateral damage. Ultrasonically activated scalpel is one of the essential instruments which are used in laparoscopic surgery. The ultrasonic scalpel is the descendant of the widely used Cavitron Kelman phaco- emulsifier system used for performing cataract surgeries. Ultrasonically activated scalpel is based on the mechanical propagation of sound or pressure waves from an active energy source to the tissues through an active blade element. Energy is supplied to either by piezoelectric or magnetic transducer which converts the electric energy or magnetic field to mechanical energy. This energy can be used for cutting and coagulation of tissue.

The ultrasonic scalpel, which is available in the market as Harmonic Scalpel®, Lotus®, SonoSurg®, etc. is composed of a generator, a hand piece and an active blade. The generator device is a microprocessor which converts the AC into a high frequency operating current at 55,000 cycles per second. Besides providing a constant high frequency it also monitors the circuit constantly like the new generation of bipolar electric devices and breaks it whenever the delivered energy is below standards set for the generator by an inbuilt feedback system. This energy is transferred to the transducer through a high conductivity cable. The transducer houses a number of piezoelectric ceramic plates bound under pressure between

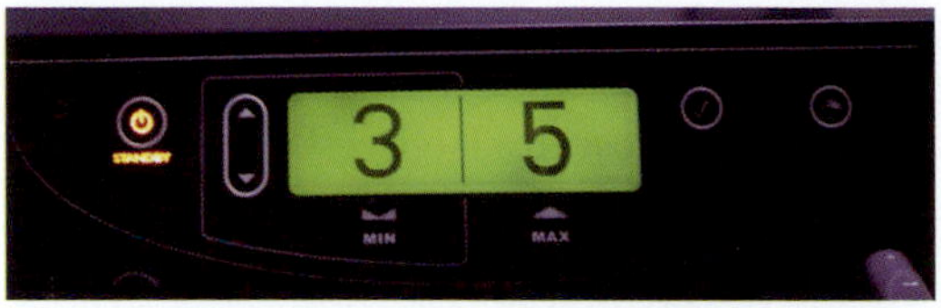

Figure 19.2: Ultrasonic generator

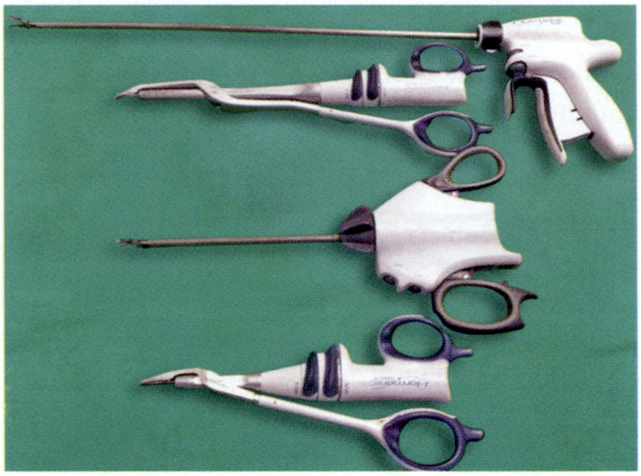

Figure 19.3: Different probes of ultrasonically activated scalpel

two metal plates. The metal plate is connected to a mount which is further attached to the blade extender and the blade. As the power is delivered to and fro motion of the crystals is transmitted to the active blade which rests in close proximity to the passive blade. This way the entire system uniformly vibrates at 55 kHz with the blade displacing longitudinally by about 60–100 micrometers.

Mechanism of Action

The transfer of mechanical energy breaks the tertiary hydrogen bonds in the tissues and generates heat from internal cellular friction. Coaptation of vessels by tamponading occurs along with sealing by denatured protein coagulum. Vibrating protein further produces secondary heating which seals larger coapted vessels. Heat, pressure and turbulence generate bubbles in tissues with high water content leading to disruption. Another mechanism of cutting is by the movement of the blade to and fro causing stretch of tissue beyond its elastic limit leading to breakage of molecular bands. This effect is more prominent in areas of high protein density like collagen rich areas. The cavitation effect occurs ahead of the blade which facilitates dissection and makes it more precise. The whole apparatus is housed in sheaths of varying lengths and diameters. The ultrasonic scalpel can coagulate blood vessels in the range of 5 mm without difficulty. The new versions of these probes, e.g. ACE, can be used to coagulate vessels up to 6–7 mm in diameter. The laparoscopic variants of the ultrasonic scalpel have a vibrating blade with sharp and blunt edges which rests along with a passive tissue pad between which the tissue is grasped and coagulated. This allows the unsupported tissue also to be coagulated with ease and without bleeding.

The propagation of sound waves though tissues which cause lower heat generation compared to electrocautery and laser devices prevents lateral damage to the surrounding structures. Charring and blackening of tissue occur at high thermal damage and are accompanied by carbonisation and smoke generation. The ultrasonic scalpel does not reach such temperatures. Ultrasonically activated scalpel works by coaptation of vessel for sealing the two walls together and forming a protein coagulum within. Electrocautery, on the other hand, causes direct thermal damage. The luminal contents on application of conventional electrocautery act as a heat sink causing one side to coagulate more than the other with resultant increase in bleeding from one wall of the vessel. The random burning of tissues by lateral thermal damage causes more difficult differentiation of planes and forms a hard eschar. The tissues thus heal poorly with more adhesion formation. There is concomitant sealing of vessels and lymphatics on using the ultrasonic scalpel through loose tissues like fat which leads to better sealing of lymphatics and haemostasis. There is also no risk of muscle or nerve stimulation by transmitted sound energy.

Besides its own advantages the ultrasonically activated shears keep the surgeon at bay from the ill effects of free current like stray electric current injuries, pad grounding problems, bowel electric injury and burns. The visual field which is crucial particularly in laparoscopic surgeries is also disturbed less with the ultrasonic shears at work, since less temperature production causes little smoke and minimal obscuration of the surgical field with tissue fog. With the back of the passive blade blunt dissection is also possible side by side with making planes. Ultrasonic devices have also found favour amongst patients with pacemakers. The theoretical advantages of the ultrasonic scalpel have been put to test by number of surgeons all across the globe with encouraging results.

MICROWAVES

Microwave energy produced through a generator (usually 0.9 to 2.45 GHz) produces heat by generation of friction by the movement of water molecules. This energy is applied to the tissue by the means of 14 G microwave antenna which is placed directly into the tumour. This antenna transmits electromagnetic waves that have been produced by the generator. These waves cause the agitation of water in and around the tissue causing coagulation and necrosis due to production of heat by friction, reaching temperatures above 55°C. Microwaves can be applied in a fashion similar to radiofrequency ablation using percutaneous, laparoscopic or open approach. Liver, lung, renal, adrenal and bone tumours have been treated with the use of microwave technology with encouraging results. Microwave generators have reduced in size considerably and have made this technology more portable. Microwave ablation carries the same advantages and disadvantages as radiofrequency ablation but cause lesser tissue charring.

CRYOABLATION

Cryoablation is a process of inducing tissue death by rapid cooling. It has become a standard modality of treatment for management of solid organ tumours and superficial lesions. Cryoablation works by intracellular crystallisation of the tissue to which it is applied and also by damaging the vasculature by forming thrombi and inducing a state of ischaemia. A second wave of reperfusion injury damages the left overs. This can be achieved by utilising a 14–16 G probe similar to the ones used with microwave and radiofrequency ablation but with different internal structure. The third generation system utilises rapidly flowing gases like carbon dioxide and argon at extremely low temperatures that cause rapid cooling of tissue to as low as –40°C. Probes can achieve temperatures close to –200°C although such temperatures are rarely used *in vivo*. After a rapid freezing cycle the tissue is left to thaw actively or passively. Thawing is important for inducing damage by restoring blood supply and allowing reperfusion injury to set in. After a slow thaw phase the whole cycle is repeated to increase effectiveness of cryoablation. Nearby important tissues are protected using a warming device intraluminally. With the use of multitine cryoablation wherein multiple small probes are used, every nook and corner of the tumour can be covered.

Advantages of cryoablation over other minimally invasive and percutaneous therapies is the ability to monitor the ice ball formed by ultrasound or direct visualisation when applied in a laparoscopic or open surgical setting. Therefore, a complete coverage of tumour can be ensured. It causes minimal pain and morbidity and is used as an office procedure in various settings. The application of probes near large vessels can cause a heat sink effect and is therefore ineffective in such lesions which lie adjacent to vessels like the renal hilum. Compared to open surgery these minimally invasive methods have a higher chance of recurrence. However, the ability to utilise them again and again gives a little advantage in this situation.

Combinations of various energy sources is mostly used for haemostasis and dissection utilising the better of every available device to deliver the best results. Some devices like the Thunderbeat® incorporate both bipolar electric energy and ultrasonic energy in one applicator and either can be used to dissect without switching instruments. It is the experience and skill of the surgeon along with the awareness regarding these new devices which ultimately delivers. Application of the right source at the right place is what makes a difference.

Key Points

1. Bipolar impedance devices, e.g. Ligasure® work on principal of impedance monitoring and feedback regulation of current.
2. Use of bipolar impedance devices prevents lateral spread of current and minimises thermal damage to surrounding tissues.
3. Radiofrequency ablation device generates temperature above 50°C when applied for more than 3 minutes by use of high frequency alternating current and induces coagulative necrosis.
4. Ultrasonically activated scalpel works on the mechanical propagation of sound or pressure waves from an active energy source to the tissues through an active blade element.
5. Cryoablation is being increasingly used for management of early solid organ tumours.

Index

Page numbers followed by *f* refer to figure

F

G

H

I

R

S

T